W9-BIF-007

Fitness Unleashed is, no pun intended, a step-by-step fitness guide for pets and people. Inspired by the *People and Pets Exercising Together* program of Hill's Pet Nutrition, and validated by research, this manual is approved by top veterinarians and human doctors as a fun, smart, sensible plan for both pets and people to lose weight, gain health and feel more alive. As a runner myself, I encourage you to take your pet to your veterinarian and also visit your doctor if you have any health concerns, then leash up your dog and step out the door to a happier, healthier, fuller life.

Daniel S. Aja, DVM
2005/2006 President
American Animal Hospital Association

To help enrich and lengthen the special relationships between people and their pets.

–Hill's Mission Statement

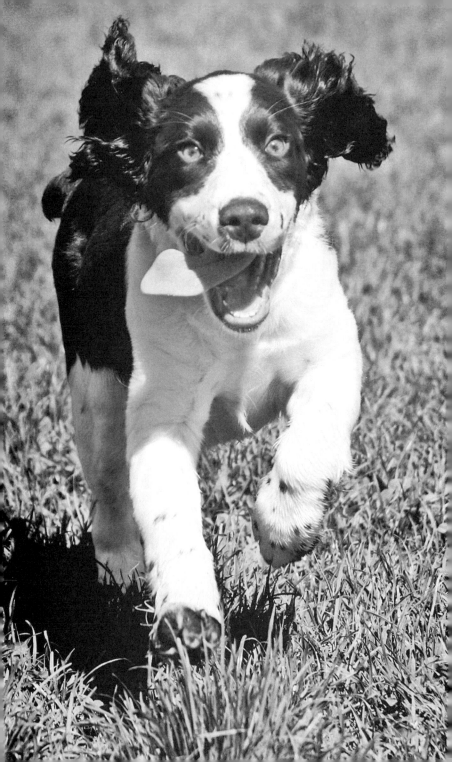

fitness
unleashed!

A Dog and Owner's Guide to
Losing Weight and Gaining
Health Together

Marty Becker, DVM, and
Robert Kushner, MD

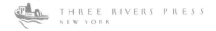

THREE RIVERS PRESS
NEW YORK

Photography credits

Photographs on pages 2, 56 © Galina Barskaya; pages 14, 31, 38, 46, 78, 117, 122, 126, 132, 137, 143–145, 167–169, 174 © Drexel Love; page 18 © Catherine Lall; page 22 © Aaron Whitney; pages 10, 29, 47 © Steven Kushner; page 42 © Sue McDonald; page 48 © Kimber Rey Solana; page 50 © Nir Alon; pages 54, 80 © First Class Photos PTY LTD; page 61 © Jose Gil; page 69 © Jose Gough; page 82 courtesy of Hill's Pet Nutrition; page 88 © George Lee; page 98 © Philip Date; page 107 © Andre Klopper; page 116 courtesy of Premier Pet Products; page 127 © WizData, Inc.; page 128 © Costin Cojocaru; page 136 © Ingvald Kaldhussater; page 140 © Joyce Sherwin; pages 158, 170 © Vendla Stockdale; page 166 © Jenny Horne; page 177 © Frances L. Fruit; page 181 © Andrew Taylor; page 185 © Ken Drori; page 190 © Fernando Castellanos.

This book is not a substitute for seeing a doctor or a veterinarian. Please consult with health-care professionals before engaging in any strenuous physical activity.

Published in the United States by Three Rivers Press, an imprint of the Crown Publishing Group, a division of Random House, Inc., New York. www.crownpublishing.com

THREE RIVERS PRESS and the Tugboat design are registered trademarks of Random House, Inc.

Library of Congress Cataloging-in-Publication Data

Becker, Marty, 1954–
Fitness unleashed: a dog and owner's guide to losing weight and gaining health/ Marty Becker and Robert Kushner.
Includes bibliographic references.
1. Physical fitness. 2. Weight loss. 3. Dog owners—Health and hygiene. 4. Dogs—Health. I. Kushner, Robert F., 1953–. II Title.

| RA781.B393 | 2006 |
| 613.7'12—dc22 | 2006000855 |

ISBN-13: 978-0-307-33858-7
ISBN-10: 0-307-33858-4

Printed in the United States of America

Design by Maggie Hinders

10 9 8 7 6 5 4 3 2
First Edition

*This book is dedicated to dog lovers everywhere
who harness the unconditional love, legendary loyalty,
and unbridled joy of the family dog, and
have seen their health directly improved as a result.
We also dedicate this book to the dogs who
have added years to our lives and life to our years.
And finally, to the veterinary and medical professionals
who with competence and compassion work
to give their clients and patients the proven tools
to lose weight, gain health, and feel more alive!*

author's note

When we read about dogs in books and magazines, they're often referenced with the pronoun "it." As animal lovers in general, and our pets' dads specifically, we didn't have the heart to use the same term that would correctly apply to a rock or a refrigerator when talking about living, breathing, tail-wagging dogs. In the following pages, dogs are generically referred to as "he." We hope all the beautiful female collies, corgis, cocker spaniels, and friends will understand this was a matter of simplicity and not in any way a slight to their sex.

acknowledgments

Please indulge us with a pun as we thank the "pack" of people who helped make *Fitness Unleashed* possible.

While we doctors with stereotypically bad handwriting are experienced enough to write a book between patient visits, for this joint project we had the good sense to enlist the help of a gifted writer, Jana Murphy. With top-notch reporting and research, Jana helped us find a perfect blending of our voices and create a book that showcases both the science and soul of unleashing fitness. Our experience in working with her was a joy.

From the first time we met our editor, Aliza Fogelson, at Clarkson Potter, we felt a connection. While she came across as knowledgeable and brainy, it was her warmth and passion for the book's premise that drew us to her. We're grateful for her calm, intelligent encouragement and direction throughout the process of creating the book.

Thanks to our peerless agents, Elisa Petrini and David Vigliano of Vigliano Associates, who helped guide us from proposal to deal to finished book.

We are especially grateful to the veterinarians, medical doctors, behaviorists, dog owners, and exercise experts and enthusiasts who shared their time, expertise, and stories with us.

We couldn't have completed this book without the support of our families, whose love for us and tolerance for the grueling hours we spent staring at the evolving chapters on a computer screen gave us the proverbial "inspiration for the perspiration."

While Marty wants to especially thank his beloved wife, Teresa, two-legged children Mikkel and Lex, and four-legged kids Quixote and Shakira, he also wants to thank Dr. Kushner's wife, Nancy, who helped behind the scenes almost daily. You won't see her name on the cover but you'll see her input on many of the pages.

Robert would also like to thank the team at Hills Pet Nutrition who sponsored the PPET (People and Pets Exercising Together) trial; registered dietitian Dawn Jackson Blatner (D.J. Blatner), who was instrumental in conducting the trial; the PPET study participants and dogs, without whom there would be no *Fitness Unleashed*; Dr. Mike Zhang, president of Diet.com, for his invaluable insight and expertise; his wife, Nancy, who has been a resourceful contributor to the project from the very beginning; his children, Sarah and Steve; and his newest four-legged addition, Cooper, who each day adds joy to the family.

Finally, a whole-hearted thank-you to the wacky, wonderful, wise pets who give us the motivation to exercise regularly (and in Dr. Kushner's case, to exercise even more), and who have graced us with the special gifts of love, loyalty, and laughter.

contents

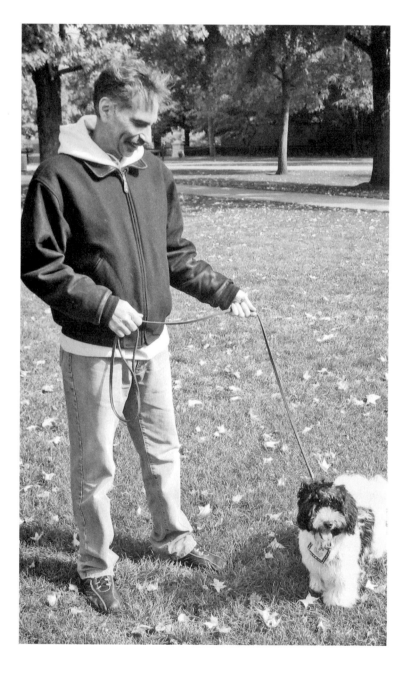

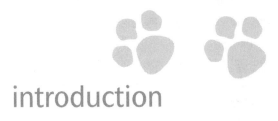

introduction

Look at Your Dog. . . .

Man's best friend? Furry foot warmer? Canine couch potato?

How about just a very good buddy who needs to lose a few pounds and needs your help to do it?

If your dog is overweight, he's in great company—according to recent studies, approximately 40 percent of pet dogs are overweight or obese. That's close to thirty million dogs in the United States alone dealing with the health implications of weight problems—symptoms like diabetes, heart problems, aching joints, difficulty breathing, intolerance of exercise, even an increased risk of cancer.

Of course, the trend toward weight gain in dogs comes directly on the heels of the same tendency among people. The percentage of the U.S. population that is overweight or obese has climbed steadily over the past decade—so much so that many medical professionals agree our collective weight problem is the number-one health concern in our society today.

When we decided to write *Fitness Unleashed*, we hoped to offer one viable solution to these two intertwined health epidemics. Our research, our instincts, and the people who have come forward to thank us on behalf of themselves and their dogs tell us we were on the right track. Fitness Unleashed is a program that builds on the wonderful, powerful bond between people and pets, and because it's constructed around that supportive, enjoyable relationship, it brings up positive associations in both two-legged and four-legged participants. We've been hearing responses to the program such as, "I never stuck to any exercise routine before—but I've kept at it because I love spending this time with my dog"; "I thought my dog was lying around and sore when he moved because he was getting old, but now he's acting like a puppy again. He was just carrying around too much 'extra baggage' "; and "Undertaking this program with my dog has made us both happier and healthier. On the days when I don't want to do it for myself, I go ahead and do it for her."

As a medical doctor and a veterinarian, we love seeing and hearing about people and pets achieving better health by taking care of each other. *Fitness Unleashed* will show you exactly how to undertake a safe, effective program that will help both you and your dog to lose weight, gain health, increase your vitality, and strengthen the bond between you.

You owe it to yourself—and to your canine best friend—to take this opportunity to do something great for both of you.

PART I

Tackling Two
Health Epidemics,
One **Leash** and
Two **Patients**
at a Time

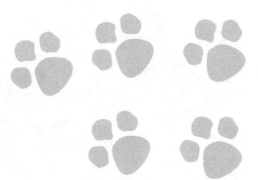

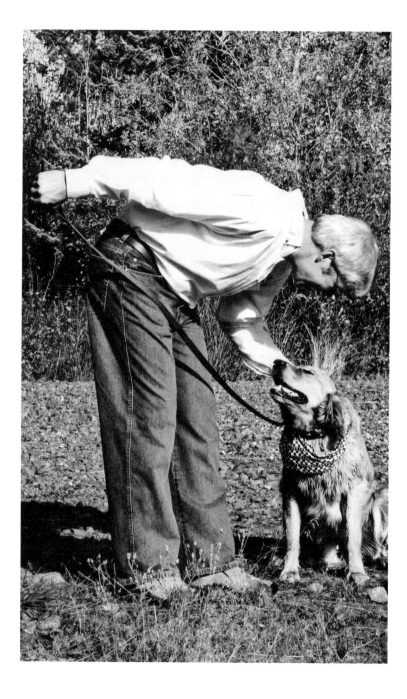

CHAPTER 1

The People and Pets Health Connection

People and dogs have always leaned on one another. In return for food, shelter, and affection, dogs are helpmates in everything from retrieving downed ducks to guarding the house and guiding the blind. For most of us, though, the "services" we receive from our dogs are much less utilitarian but equally endearing: they adore us when we're up, when we're down, and even when we're having a bad hair day, wearing our rattiest old bathrobe, and feeling cranky. They sit on (not just at) our feet, wait for us at the door, and go to great lengths to wriggle into a spot right beside us whenever they can get away with it. They make us laugh by being silly and full of puppy charm, regardless of their age; and they have an uncanny ability to read our emotions and sync themselves up, ready and willing to be cheerful or mad just because we are.

Somehow all the small acts of affection, concern, loyalty, and furriness add up to more than just gestures and companionship. Research has proven that having a dog is good for your health in a number of measurable and not-so-measurable ways. Studies show that people who own pets tend to have lower blood pressure and lower cholesterol levels than those who don't. Pet owners have better odds of surviving heart attacks than patients without pets. As a group, pet owners find their chronic pain diminished, make fewer trips to the doctor, are less medicated, less lonely, less depressed, and less stressed than their petless counterparts—and those are just the subtle, unintended benefits of time spent with our four-legged and furry companions. For those who deliberately harness the health benefits of pets, there are even greater rewards to be reaped. Dogs have been trained to provide services that assist people with a vast range of needs—including guiding the blind, serving as hearing companions for the deaf, helping the physically challenged to overcome obstacles, and serving to alert their owners of imminent seizures or blood-sugar imbalances. Dogs are used to tremendous effect in therapeutic and educational settings, doing everything from helping kids learn to read in classrooms to providing much-needed inspiration for residents of nursing homes to increase their levels of activity and social interaction.

In these kinds of win/win partnerships, dogs also reap some surprising benefits. You may have read that when you pet your dog, your blood pressure drops and the level of the feel-good hormones such as oxytocin, prolactin, and serotonin in your blood increases. But did you also know that during that interaction, your dog experiences the same benefits—*his* blood pressure drops and he receives a biochemical spa treatment, too? Your dog's longevity is directly tied to the care you provide; everything from a roof over his head at night and regular veterinary visits to optimum nutrition and the affection that makes him feel loved and needed contributes to his good health. A dog who's been abandoned has a life expectancy of a year or less. Those who live in loving homes can expect to live to their breeds' expectancy—anywhere from seven years to eighteen or more.

As a group, pet owners find their chronic pain diminished, make fewer trips to the doctor, are less medicated, less lonely, less depressed, and less stressed than their petless counterparts—and those are just the subtle, unintended benefits of time spent with our four-legged and furry companions.

Despite all the good that people and pets do one another, in recent years our healthful relationship has taken an unexpected turn. In our increasingly sedentary, stressed-out, and overfed culture, people are consuming more calories, exercising less, and collectively getting more overweight by the minute. Without intending to cause any harm, many of us have shared our generous portions and inactive routines with our beloved pets. We share our couches and beds, as well as our ice cream and cookies, with our dogs, and they're very happy to get on board with whatever lifestyle we're offering—especially one that's heavy on the treats. Centuries of species self-preservation have left most dogs with a strong desire to consume any edible bite they can find—they've historically survived as scavengers, after all. Many will eat as much, and as often, as you'll let them.

Scaling Up, Side by Side

ONE big (and growing) result of these changes in lifestyle for pets and people is the effect Dr. Kushner has dubbed *scaling up*—weight gain that's a common, if unwelcome, life experience. Scaling up describes how people put on pounds not just through failed willpower or the wrong mix of carbs and protein, but because we live in a society where every aspect of our food consumption and activity levels seems designed to add weight to our frames. Factors like crammed-full schedules, crammed-full plates, desk jobs, slowing metabolisms, and a lack of time to devote to the care and maintenance of our bodies all contribute to it gradually. Scaling up doesn't even necessarily imply poor choices—it means that just following the basic eating and exercise trends our society offers is enough to make trying to maintain—or reduce—your current weight a losing battle.

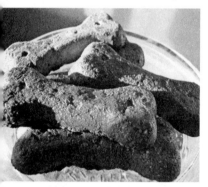

The concept applies equally well to dogs, who are truly the victims of their environments as they pack on the pounds. Often, it's just our generosity that's making them chubby! Our food-is-love affection adds up to lots of treats, lots of off-the-table snacks, and too much kibble in the bowl from day to day.

Surprisingly, when you look past the basic calories-in/calories-out equation for both people and dogs, the roots of this crisis are very similar for both species. In a nutshell: most of us are not using our bodies the way nature—and natural selection—intended. The human body is "designed" for function—for movement. Up until the twentieth-century inventions of the automobile, the washing machine, riding lawnmowers, power tools, personal computers, and countless other gadgets and gizmos designed to reduce the physical labor in our personal and professional lives, average folks were in near-constant motion. A recent study that highlighted this point was led by researchers from the University of Tennessee. To try to come up with an assessment of the physical exertion previous generations might have made, the team asked members of an old-order Amish community in Canada to wear pedometers as they went about their daily lives. The chosen community is one that shuns modern conveniences and continues to maintain a self-sufficient farming lifestyle. Though there was no deliberate effort made by the participants to "exercise," as they kept up their normal routines, the men logged an

EVERYDAY SCALING-UP FACTORS

FOR PEOPLE

Restaurant portions—It's not uncommon to find that one plateful of food at a restaurant contains a full day's worth of calories. (For example, an order of Chili's ribs contains just under 1,200 calories—without any side dishes or drinks; ditto for half of a rotisserie chicken from Boston Market, a stuffed chicken marsala entrée at Olive Garden, or just half of a Bloomin' Onion at the Outback.)

Portions at home—The occasional gut-busting restaurant meal wouldn't really have significant health implications for most of us if it weren't for the fact that the portion explosion has somehow found its way into our homes. According to a Tufts University report, in the past twenty years Americans have taken to eating twenty-two more calorie's worth of dessert at every meal and making burgers, pasta, and cookie servings nearly twice as big as we used to. Even the average empty plate for sale is bigger than it was fifteen years ago.

"Low fat" and "low carb," but not all that low cal—Foods labeled with assorted "lows" have become increasingly popular, but they're also widely misused because buyers tend to think it's okay to eat more and to eat more often.

Liquid calories—With a can of Coke containing 140 calories, and the average mocha latte or vanilla chai containing 220 or more, it's far too easy to rack up a wealth of calories in drinks alone.

Stress, stress, and more stress—The problem with following any diet plan is that everyday life gets in the way. The stress, obstacles, barriers, priorities, and other responsibilities in life typically trump one's best intentions. It's a common situation, especially among adults with families to care for, because by the time every spouse-, child-, and work-related priority has been attended to, there's barely enough time left for a shower, let alone a workout.

Driving destinations—Once upon a time, long, long ago, when a person wanted to visit a friend, buy a pound of coffee, see the doctor, or visit the park, those things were done under the person's own steam. In some urban centers, this is still the case, although taking a cab or a bus to go a few blocks isn't uncommon. But in our age of urban—and suburban—sprawl, each of those things is frequently accomplished by driving instead. According to the Centers for Disease Control (CDC), the number of trips Americans made by walking declined 40 percent between 1977 and 1995.

Less and less leisure time—Research suggests that the average American has picked up a longer work week and a longer commute over the past thirty years—and in the process lost more than 30 percent of his or her leisure time. Having less time to pick and choose our own activities likely contributes to the fact that most of us aren't finding enough time to exercise.

Surf and screen—According to Nielsen Media Research, the average American watches about four hours of television per day, and in addition, many of us spend substantial blocks of free time staring at computer screens. All those hours frittered away in front of screens may contribute to our societal scaling up more than any other single factor.

FOR DOGS
Canine cookies, biscuits, and treats galore—Who'd have thought it was even possible to have so many varieties on the once-basic dog biscuit? Today, not only do we have Snausages and Beggin' Strips and Scooby Snacks (and dogs who know darn well which are their fa-

vorites), we've even got doggy bakeries with homemade carob cookies, puppy pizzas, and birthday cakes!

The trickle-down portion effect—We've all been there ourselves: either you or a family member notes that it just doesn't seem fair that the people in the family can have a full plate of, say, spaghetti and meatballs, when all Rover gets is just that wee little bowl of dog food. Moments later, said family pooch is either (a) dining on a substantially bigger serving of the usual chow or (b) happily gulping down the normal portion—topped with a hearty helping of spaghetti on top. Our families could have succumbed to this, too, but as a veterinarian and an obesity expert, we know full well that this kind of logic makes Fido momentarily happy only at the long-term expense of his health and his waistline.

A life of leisure—Gone are the days when most family dogs had to earn their keep. At the same time your own work week is getting longer, at least statistically speaking, many dogs' resting hours are growing by equal proportion. While "the boss" is keeping long hours at the office, many of our dogs are snoozing away the hours with nothing but snuggling the couch cushions and mangling the occasional slipper to keep them occupied—certainly no activity strenuous enough to burn off that bowl of spaghetti.

Spaying/Neutering—One of the great achievements of the past two decades for the veterinary community and for animal shelters and animal lovers has been the increased practice of spaying and neutering pets. This is important to dogs everywhere, as there are still so many who don't have the comfort of safe, loving homes. Unfortunately, though, many dog owners are never told that spaying or neutering reduces a dog's need for calories by about 5 percent. Most keep the diet the same, and find that the dog gets bigger.

average of more than 18,000 steps a day. The women logged an average of more than 14,000. To put those numbers in perspective, the average American is currently walking between 3,000 and 5,000 steps a day, and the goal you'll read about in this book, the one fitness plans and gurus across the country have embraced as an ideal exertion level, is 10,000 steps. Taking close to double that number of steps, the Amish men were getting the same level of workout as a long-distance runner by doing just their daily work. Though their other physical efforts were not measured, it's a pretty safe bet that the people in this community were also doing more lifting, bending, squatting, stretching, and general exercising than your average, say, computer programmer, magazine editor, or retail-store clerk.

Just as we humans are not living up to our physical potential, neither are our dogs. Before selective breeding, rather than finding food in a bowl, they were always walking and running in search of "fast food." In more recent history, hundreds of years of selective breeding designed most dogs to be tireless physical workers. Breeds like Labs and goldens and border collies and shelties and huskies and many, many others are genetically programmed to run, not just walk, for hours without getting worn out. Historically, the majority of dog

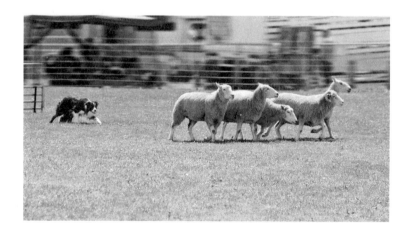

breeds were selectively bred to either hunt or herd alongside their owners. Their functions ranged widely, but in most cases, the intent was to train an effective "tool" for the family. Everything about their frames, their musculature, and their mental abilities is designed for a life on the go. It contradicts your dog's hardwiring and natural inclinations to sideline all that physicality on the couch, often alone, day in and day out, not far from pantries bursting with food and treats. As both species become more and more out of shape, we experience almost identical health complications of overweight and obesity, including heart disease, diabetes, joint ailments, and an increased risk of cancer. New studies even suggest those extra pounds may put us at higher risk for Alzheimer's disease as well. What's more, we share the experience of getting trapped by our own symptoms—the more weight we gain, the more the aches and pains and feelings of being tired and heavy keep us from getting the exercise that could help improve our circumstances.

Why Worry?

IN our "thin is in" culture, with underweight models and actors staring back at us from every billboard, magazine cover, TV, and computer screen, most people with weight issues are aware of the problem. If you have any doubt, it's easy to find a Body Mass Index (BMI) chart and a scale to make an assessment. (For convenience we've added a BMI chart with some examples on page 204.) For better or worse, that's not at all the case for assessing the body condition of dogs. Because of substantial breed differences, nailing down pet-weight statistics is sticky business. Depending on the source, the number of dogs that are overweight or obese is about 40 percent and rising steadily. One recent study (of both dogs and cats) puts the number as high as 60 percent. Even more surprising is the fact that almost half of the owners of overweight pets that participated in that study described their pets' body condition as "ideal."

The perception of pudgy pooches as perfectly fine is one of the significant challenges pet owners and veterinarians face in trying to help dogs maintain healthy weights. We really do love them just the way they are, and there are no rail-thin dog models reminding us at our every turn that our pups might have a problem. As the study mentioned in the previous paragraph shows, we not only love our dogs at any weight or size, we're often oblivious to the fact that there's anything "wrong" with them at all.

So, if your dog is happy carrying around a few extra pounds, and if you adore him at any weight, why bother to help him get in shape? The fact is that overweight pets cope with almost all the same health implications that overweight people do—but they cope with them sooner and with more potential ill effects. Dogs don't have the luxury of long lives to cushion the complications of weight gain. While you have a projected lifespan of seven decades plus a few years, your dog is looking at a much shorter life. With an average of twelve short years on this earth, dogs truly need every health advantage they can get. Research shows that trim pets live about 15 percent longer, or an average of two additional years, than overweight pets. That's an incredibly sobering statistic for anyone who lives with and loves a dog. The fountain of youth for our furry friends may just be putting less food in their mouths and more miles on their feet.

With an average of twelve short years on this earth, dogs truly need every health advantage they can get. Research shows that trim pets live about 15 percent longer, or an average of two additional years, than overweight pets.

BY THE BREED

Any dog can eat too much and not exercise enough and gain weight, but there are a handful of breeds that really have to watch their waistlines, so to speak. Just as heredity plays a significant part in the risk for weight problems in people, it also does in dogs. In fact, as much as 70 percent of the risk for becoming overweight in dogs may be attributable to breed. Think about it: when was the last time you saw a chubby greyhound? How about a chubby Labrador retriever (or, as veterinarians commonly call them out of earshot of their owners, flabrador retrievers)?

Labrador retrievers, Cairn terriers, cocker spaniels, dachshunds, corgis, shelties, basset hounds, beagles, and King Charles spaniels are all prone to putting on extra weight. Luckily, they're all great candidates for a walking-with-you program, too.

The effect of extra weight on a dog's lifespan carries across breeds, affecting dogs as different from one another as bichons and beagles and boxers. There is another big consideration to keep in mind when you assess your dog's weight, though, and that's his size. On a body frame that averages 150 pounds, humans have a little room to grow, so to speak. But small dogs begin to suffer health problems with just a couple extra pounds on their compact bodies. In fact, just 1 extra pound on the frame of a 10-pound dog is equivalent to more than 20 pounds on an average adult human! If you think that an extra pound on Fido is no big deal, just put a can of soup on the middle of your pet's back, and imagine him packing it around 24/7.

A New Solution

UNTIL now, the weight-related health crisis in people and the same crisis in dogs have been addressed separately. Veterinarians recommend diet changes and increased activity for overweight dogs. Doctors recommend diet changes and increased activity for overweight people. For some, those suggestions, or one of a host of programs designed to help them stick to the changes, help solve the problem. For many, the challenge is more than they're ready to face. Many dog owners even tell us they aren't able to stick to their *dogs'* weight-loss programs because they can't stand to see their four-legged friends deprived. (If you've ever watched your dog put on a full-fledged, Oscar-worthy "Can't you see I'm wasting away?" routine to get a scrap of food, you can understand how this could happen.) The challenge, of course, is figuring out a way to change our eating and exercise habits without making our lives so miserable that we give up and quit before the program can make any difference.

The solution comes in the form of Fitness Unleashed, a simple, comprehensive program that encourages dog owners to harness the inspiration, companionship, and sense of duty to their friend by turning to the four-legged personal trainer who works just for the love of it. The National Institutes of Health estimates that Americans spend $36 billion a year on weight-loss products and services, but for many of us, the best piece of exercise equipment is standing by the door with its leash in its mouth, with no membership fees or installment payments required.

The Fitness Unleashed program came about when a research study caused our professional paths to cross. As authors and guardians of health, both of us have built our careers on promoting health and well-being—in people, in pets, and now in both. In our separate fields, we've kept our eyes and ears open for methods, ideas, and innovations that might make life easier or more enjoyable for the patients who rely on us. One eye-opening, ear-perking moment occurred three years ago when an executive from Hill's Pet Nutrition called Dr. Kushner to propose jointly developing a weight-management program that would help both overweight people and pets. With so many proven, positive health implications of pets in other areas of medicine, it was a concept that made perfect sense. After all, many weight-loss studies had shown that social support for any diet and exercise program is one of the best predictors of its success. Having someone around to encourage you to stick with it, to participate alongside you, and to push you through the hard days is one of the true keys to successful weight loss. Why not take a hard look at how a group of overweight pet owners and their overweight dogs might be able to help each other shed pounds and gain health?

Both Dr. Kushner and Hill's Pet Nutrition were interested to see if a study could prove dogs were as good at providing social support as people are. If it worked, a whole new type of fitness program might be possible.

Dr. Kushner designed the study to include a group of overweight dog owners and their overweight dogs and a group of overweight people who didn't have dogs. He called it People and Pets Exercising Together, or PPET. Hill's agreed to fund and support it. Surprisingly, recruitment began slowly. Neither group that had been asked to look for possible candidates wanted to risk insulting any patients by asking if they'd like to participate in a study for people with a weight problem, an approach in keeping with much of the medical and veterinary communities' determination to ignore the epidemic in the room.

When PPET got under way, however, at Northwestern University in Chicago, the differences in the two groups, each of which were receiving both nutritional and exercise counseling, were in small, surprising things. Both groups steadily changed their eating and exercise habits and lost weight, which was expected with the close supervision and coaching. The dogs, who were fed Hill's Prescription Diet Canine r/d food and prescribed exercise, also lost effectively. What was not expected was that the dog owners rarely complained about their exercise assignments—which all pertained to working out with their dogs. In weekly meetings about the program, the dog owners routinely focused not on their own weight loss, which was significant, but on the positive changes they were seeing in their dogs' health. The dog owners bonded with one another at these meetings in a way the research team hadn't seen coming. They shared stories about their dogs, joked with one another about which dog could beg the most effectively and about which dogs had the most weight to lose. They celebrated unexpected milestones together—things like the first time the dog chased them around the house, leash in mouth, insistent on a walk; or the first time they realized the dog was bounding, not dragging himself, up a flight of stairs, thanks to significant weight loss.

In an undertaking that is almost always (and necessarily) self-focused, these people were all enthusiastic about doing something that helped them bond with and benefit their dogs. Their exit interviews at the end of the study were all about their dogs, with the recurring theme that they stuck to it because the dogs loved it.

Since the results of the PPET study were announced, they've inspired an incredible spate of publicity—media outlets ranging from the *New York Times* to *Dog Fancy* have reported on this nontraditional approach to weight loss. The publicity, and the resulting contacts we've had with dog owners everywhere we go, continues to confirm what we've believed all along: millions of people who are looking for a safe, healthy way to lose extra weight and help their beloved hounds lose some pounds can find a program they can not only live with, but learn to love. It's as simple as following the guidelines we've laid out in the coming chapters of *Fitness Unleashed*.

MEET THE DOCTOR

When I was growing up, I always wanted to be a doctor. After medical school, I teamed up with a registered dietitian and opened a practice that specialized in helping overweight patients lose pounds and reclaim their health. It was a fairly new area of specialization, but with my interest in nutrition science, it seemed like the right fit.

Once the practice was opened, we waited for the patients to come. I remember in those early days, more than twenty years ago, literally gazing out the window or stepping into the hall to look at the people passing by, thinking, "There must be *someone* out there who needs this kind of help."

Times have certainly changed. Today, the majority of Americans are overweight or obese. In two decades of studying why our society continues to gain weight and how I can help my patients make lifestyle changes so they can lose pounds and maintain good health,

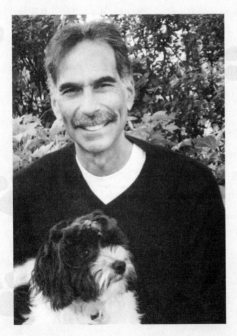

I've learned a great deal about how every aspect of our culture is increasingly pushing us toward putting on extra pounds. It's a sneaky phenomenon, because high-calorie foods, oversized portions, and constant suggestions to eat and eat more are so pervasive in our environment that it's almost impossible to escape them. Time and again I meet with patients who are successful and in control of almost every aspect of their lives—but they feel frustration and powerlessness when it comes to managing their weight.

That's why I wrote my book *The Personality Type Diet*, because I had learned that losing unwanted pounds requires a personalized program to meet each individual's needs and lifestyle. My passion to help people on a very personal level is one of the reasons I came to study how overweight dog lovers had a hidden weight-loss buddy literally right under their feet. When I conducted a weight-loss study called People and Pets Exercising Together in 2004, it was groundbreaking for pairing overweight people and their overweight pets in diet and exercise regimens. I hoped to demonstrate that a dog can offer social support to a person who is trying to change his or her lifestyle—and the study did just that. What also became apparent during the research was something I hadn't expected: the participants who followed the program with their dogs had an entirely different, much more positive experience as they successfully lost weight than the people in the control group who undertook the program alone. The pet owners laughed, they bonded with each other, they enjoyed spending time with their dogs, and—regardless of whether they'd joined the study primarily to lose pounds off their own frames or to help get their dogs in shape—they *stuck to it* month after month, and many are still sticking to it, because they genuinely enjoy the experience.

Finding a variable that brought a surprising level of comfort and even happiness to what would otherwise have been a test of participants' willpower and determination was the inspiration for this book and the starting point for Fitness Unleashed.

MEET THE VETERINARIAN

My entire career has been built on my unwavering belief that pets don't just make people feel good, but that they actually *are* good for us, physically, emotionally, and socially. This special affection connection between pets and people, which we call *the Bond*, is inspiring, life affirming, and mutually supporting. Somehow, dogs have willingly forsaken their own species to share humans' hearts and homes. We're magically connected and better together than apart. My early veterinary practice was a departure from anything my community had previously seen because it treated every person's pet like a part of the family. I helped clients select the perfect pet, gave behavior problems just as much priority as fleas and ticks, counseled about optimum nutrition, and spent a good part of my time with my clients and patients making sure that the Bond between them was nurtured.

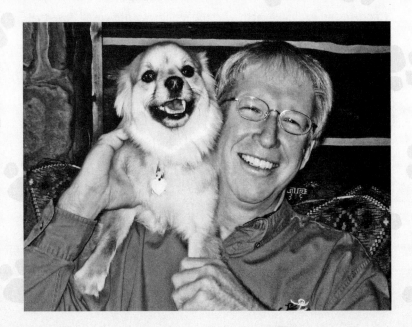

In recent years, my career has become increasingly focused on celebrating and protecting the Bond between people and pets. I've spent more and more of my time writing books, magazine articles, and newspaper columns about the power of that Bond, and I've traveled across the country and around the world to speak in person, on the radio, and to television audiences about it. That work has extended to many areas, including promoting spay/neuter campaigns and helping shed light on the plight of countless desperately needy animals in shelters. These days, I'm able to reach millions of people in the same way I had the privilege of working one on one with them in my first veterinary practice.

I've always been acutely aware of the fact that people and pets can better one another's health, but in 2002, I embarked on the research and writing of a new book titled *The Healing Power of Pets*, and was able to delve into this area and learn more than I'd imagined possible about just how symbiotic the relationship between our species is. My coauthor reminded me at the time that it was our job to prove and explain exactly why the intuitive sense we all have that pets can be good for us is, in fact, a truth.

That "prove it" mind-set was still with me when I read that Dr. Kushner's PPET study was under way, and I knew instantly that I'd found a terrific ally. It has been a privilege to team up with this new partner as we've worked together to create a fitness program—and a fitness mentality—that equally benefits people and dogs. Fitness Unleashed is a program that any medical doctor, any veterinarian, and anyone who owns and loves a dog can wrap their arms around. It's as great an incarnation of the powerful Bond between people and pets as any I've ever seen.

A DOG-GONE GREAT IDEA

Just how smart and sensible is dog walking as a weight-loss, health-gain tool? We asked some of the top health, fitness, and veterinary organizations in the country (and in the world) to share their thoughts on the benefits of dog walking, and here's what we heard back from them:

American College of Sports Medicine

Of all the different pieces of exercise equipment that you can use for your health, a pair of comfortable shoes, a leash for your dog, and, of course, your dog are the very best. That's all you need to get started to enhance both your health and that of your pet. The American College of Sports Medicine (ACSM) and Centers for Disease Control recommend that you accumulate thirty minutes of physical activity on most, if not all, days of the week. Although simple, this is not an easy task for most people in our overscheduled, busy days. If you are a pet owner, your love for your pet can be your motivation to be more active. Think of how great your pet will look and feel, and then remember that we resemble our pets.

—CARL FOSTER, PhD, PRESIDENT

American College of Veterinary Internal Medicine

The health benefits of a proper diet and exercise are well known to both the practitioners of veterinary and human medicines. A simple and effective way to reduce the incidence of diseases related to obesity in our companion animals and ourselves is to adopt a regular routine of walking. "A mile a day keeps the doctor away."

—DR. MARY ROSE PARADIS, PRESIDENT

Arthritis Foundation

A brisk walk twice a day can help keep you and your dog fit while reducing arthritis pain and swelling.

—Dr. John H. Klippel, president and CEO

American Heart Association

Physical inactivity is a major risk factor for heart disease and stroke. In the United States, 250,000 deaths per year—about 12 percent of total deaths— are due to a lack of regular physical activity. The American Heart Association is trying to change that by encouraging people to get active. By doing at least thirty minutes of moderate physical activity a day you can help reduce your risk of heart disease, keep weight under control, improve blood cholesterol levels, prevent and manage high blood pressure. One of the fastest and easiest ways to get started is walking. Take a walk with your family, your friends, and your dog. Pets need exercise, too, and if that motivates you to get out and walk every day, then grab the leash and get going. Pet owners even register their dogs to participate in our annual Heart Walks nationwide. It's a great way to support the fight against heart disease and stroke and help keep your heart healthy, too.

—Robert H. Eckel, MD, president

American Council on Exercise

Walking is arguably the most popular physical activity in the United States, and for good reason. It's easy to do, inexpensive, joint friendly, and can be well tolerated by virtually everyone. A consistent walking habit conditions your heart, strengthens your bones and muscles, elevates your mood, improves your mental outlook, and reduces your risk for a variety of chronic diseases. Despite its numerous beneficial effects, many individuals find it difficult to walk on a regular basis, in part due to a lack of motivation.

In Fitness Unleashed, the authors offer the perfect remedy for the individual lacking motivation: exercise with a partner—a four-legged one, your dog. Walking your dog around the neighborhood or through a park can provide the perfect way to help you stay motivated and committed to your walking routine.

—CEDRIC X. BRYANT, PhD, FACSM, CHIEF EXERCISE
PHYSIOLOGIST/VICE PRESIDENT OF EDUCATIONAL SERVICES

American Cancer Society

Being physically active helps you look good, feel good, and can reduce your risk of cancer and other chronic diseases. Exercising with a partner can help give you the motivation you need to keep it up, and what better partner than your dog? Rain or shine, hot or cold, he's ready to go and will never oversleep or get stuck late at the office.

—COLLEEN DOYLE, MS, RD, DIRECTOR,
NUTRITION AND PHYSICAL ACTIVITY

American Animal Hospital Association

Exercise is a key ingredient in keeping your pet healthy, and walking with your dog is a great way to help keep him fit and active. This type of simple exercise will also benefit us through enhanced fitness and the development of a deeper bond with our pets.

—MICHAEL P. ANDREWS, DVM,
PRESIDENT, 2006–2007

American Veterinary Medical Association

Pet wellness promotes a long and enjoyable relationship between humans and animals. As for people, exercise is an important part of wellness, plus it has the benefit of quality time for both the two- and four-legged partners.

—BONNIE V. BEAVER, BS, DVM, MS, DIPLOMATE
ACVB, IMMEDIATE PAST PRESIDENT

The Cooper Institute

Major health organizations all over the world now recognize the importance of regular physical activity to function, health, and quality of life. The consensus recommendation for physical activity is to accumulate at least thirty minutes of moderate intensity physical activity such as walking on at least five days of the week. Note that you do not have to do the entire thirty minutes at one time. Drs. Becker and Kushner provide suggestions on how you and your dog can get regular exercise, become more fit, and reap all the benefits of regular activity. Walking your dog every day will do you both a world of good.

—STEVEN N. BLAIR, PRESIDENT AND CEO

Weight Watchers International

Having a dog has a wide range of benefits—both physical and mental. Studies have shown that having a pet may even prolong the life of the owner. And just by meeting your dog's needs, you can also meet your own need . . . for exercise, one of the key components of the Weight Watchers program. Walking your dog keeps you more physically active; helping you to stay fit and maintain a healthy weight. I know from experience: my mixed breed dog, Carmen, helps me not only get in my daily physical activity, but enjoy it, too.

—KAREN MILLER-KOVACH, MS, RD, CHIEF SCIENTIFIC
OFFICER, VICE PRESIDENT OF PROGRAM DEVELOPMENT,
WEIGHT WATCHERS INTERNATIONAL

CHAPTER 2

Why Your Dog Is the Ideal Workout Partner

Anyone who's ever tried to begin an exercise program knows that starting off and sticking to it are two entirely different challenges. Making long-term changes in our habits and routines takes substantial commitment—and there are all too many occasions that'll test it: Week 2, when your enthusiasm starts wearing off; Week 5 (or 6), when you've tasted success, then reach a plateau where the weight is sticking stubbornly; Week 8, when it's cold (or hot, or rainy) outside; Week 9, postflu.

In twenty-five years of helping his patients achieve weight-loss results, Dr. Kushner has seen hundreds of reasons—some legitimate, some not so compelling—win out over good intentions to get fit and lose weight. Over that time, in Dr. Kushner's offices and in those of weight-loss experts worldwide, one pattern that's clearly emerged among people who succeed is the presence of social support. If you have a doctor, a neighbor, a spouse, a friend, or a support group backing you up, cheering you on, and helping to keep

THE VETERINARIAN SAYS

You might call me Exhibit A in the Fitness Unleashed phenomenon. At forty-nine years old, six feet one inch tall, and an uncomfortable 236 pounds, I had come to the end of my belt. For years, I'd been loosening it, one notch after the next, moving farther past the old familiar crease in the leather. When I realized my gut had passed the point where I could cinch it at the last hole, I didn't panic—I went out to the barn, got a leather punch, and made a new hole. A couple months later, though, it had shrunk (or I had grown) again. I was beltless, toying with the idea of suspenders, thinking there was a little too much Ho! Ho! Ho! in that look for a guy who felt as young as I did.

Right around the time my belt ran out, I had another rude awakening. I have an old spinal injury that was surgically corrected when I was a little younger and thinner. At around the 230-pound mark, my body objected to having all that extra baggage on its fragile, ex-

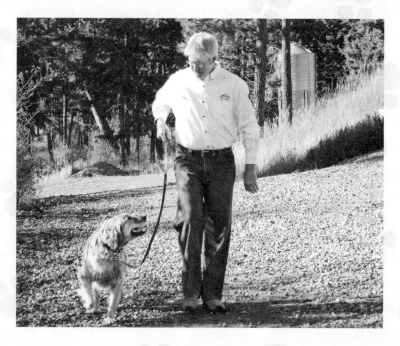

pertly, expensively protected nerve system. Once again, I started experiencing numbness down my right side. That development also got my attention.

Even more than what I saw in the mirror or what I felt in my body, though, I was concerned about what I was seeing in my wife's eyes. Teresa and I are best friends and we've been married for twenty-six years. While I have chicken winged and potato chipped myself into various states of questionable health over the years, she has exercised and eaten healthfully and, I suspect, even aged backward from time to time. Teresa would never put me down for letting my weight get away from me, but she would, and did, let me know she was worried about my health.

So there I was, uncomfortable, up two sizes, no belt, numb on my right side, my loving, worrying wife reminding me that I had a family and a career and a community that all needed me. When my daughter Mikkel challenged me to a weight-loss contest, I knew it was a bet I needed to take.

If you were to drill straight through the floor of my den, which houses a big-screen TV and my favorite couch, you'd find I have a very nice home gym, with all kinds of high-tech equipment. My family has used it well over the years. Unfortunately, I hate it. The experience of climbing on a machine and plodding along like a hamster has never appealed to me. Watching the red blinking numbers counting down the minutes of my workout, I feel like I'm just serving out a daily sentence.

Instead, I turned to our fifteen-month-old golden retriever, Shakira, for inspiration. She was at an age when dogs need all the exercise they can get—and I guess I'm at an age when guys need that, too. I figured if I could dedicate myself to walking with her every single day for long enough, I'd spare myself the misery and monotony of the treadmill (I called it the dreadmill), stair stepper (stairway to hell), and the stationary bike. I wouldn't have that nagging feeling I was turning into a step-by-Stepford husband.

Shakira and I jumped in with all six feet, walking at least thirty minutes every morning, and sometimes taking a second walk at night. Our walks never felt like punishment. I felt anticipation, rather than apathy, and though we covered at least two miles every day, I never felt like I was slogging through a workout I could do without. Starting this routine was like finding something I'd been missing all along—so much so that I'm still sticking to it. I love getting outside and feeling the jolt of the wind and the natural light—even the smack of occasional precipitation. I enjoy spending time in the company of our zany, happy, grateful dog. Even in the beginning, before I'd lost any weight, I'd come in from that walk every morning feeling healthy, invigorated, and charged up for the day.

Because I felt so good, I stuck to it, and in over six months, I lost 42 pounds. In the end, I had to buy a new belt anyway—a smaller one.

you honest, you have a better chance of success than if you go it alone.

New science, including Dr. Kushner's People and Pets Exercising Together study, shows a dog is as capable of providing needed social support as a person. Some people find canine social support to be even more effective.

To sort out exactly why and how our four-legged friends are great weight-loss partners, we interviewed dog-walking devotees from across the country in our research for *Fitness Unleashed*. Many had lost weight through exercise routines they shared with their dogs—and a surprising number had lost those pounds inadvertently: walking was something they were doing for the dog, or to relieve stress, or to get a little sunshine, and the results they found in the fit of their clothes and the face of the scale were a pleasant and welcome surprise. Even those who set out to lose weight were surprised at how painless and organic a dog-walking routine can be.

As we continue to seek explanations for how, and why, this kind of routine works, there is clearly some common ground. Here are the biggest, most compelling reasons, offered up by individuals who have all been able to successfully unleash fitness for themselves.

Elephants Aren't the Only Ones Who Never Forget!

LET'S say you start a daily walking program with your neighbor, every weekday morning at 7:30. On Monday, you meet and walk. Ditto Tuesday. Wednesday, you meet at 7:40, but still go. Thursday, it's raining, and your neighbor (or is it you?) calls to beg off. Thursday night, you check the Internet or nightly news and agree that you will be too tired or it will be too cold to go on Friday. It's a discouraging scenario, sometimes played out over more than just a week, but it's also very common. (We've done it ourselves a time or two. . . .)

A four-legged workout partner, by contrast, is one who will never, ever let you down—not even when "forgetting" about your workout is exactly what you'd like to do. With no repertoire of excuses, Rover will not decline to walk in any weather or at any level of exhaustion. He will, in fact, jump, whine, bark, wiggle, dance, engage the tail-helicopter rotor, and do whatever is necessary to drag your butt off the couch and out the door when it's time for his scheduled

A four-legged workout partner . . . is one who will never, ever let you down—not even when "forgetting" about your workout is exactly what you'd like to do.

walk. Remember, dogs have no watches, day planners, cell phones, or PDAs to track other commitments and time. Your workouts together are the highlights of their days. You can count on them daily to deliver you out the door and on your journey back to fitness.

Janet Agranoff learned all about dogs' level of determination to stick to the walking routine when she joined People and Pets Exercising Together. Janet has struggled with her weight all her life, but when her daughter, who had recently suffered the loss of someone she loved, asked with genuine concern, "Mom, could you take really, extra good care of yourself so you don't die until you get very old?" Janet decided she would try a new means of whittling away at the weight that was adversely affecting her health.

Sticking to an exercise routine and changing her eating habits were both hard, but walking Chico, her golden retriever, was easy. "We were walking thirty to forty minutes a day, and it was a pleasant time for me—much more pleasant than trying to ignore Chico's

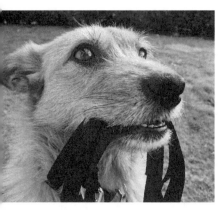

begging to get on with it," Janet explains. "I would take my kids to school, come home and have my coffee, and that's when the whining started. If we didn't go right away, he'd just torture me until I gave in and took him. It was impossible to forget. I've walked with friends before, and sooner or later one of us just stops calling, but my dog kept after me day after day."

At the end of the study, Janet had lost 10 percent of her body weight—an achievement she's been able to maintain. But it was Chico, she says, who was the "star loser." The gigantic golden was a hefty 135 pounds at his first weigh-in, and a tall, lean 100 pounds at the last.

"Before we started walking, I hadn't realized that he was so out of shape," Janet recalls with a smile. "But as the weight came off, he wanted to walk farther and longer and play more, and he started acting like a puppy again. Even if the exercise had not been so good for me, I would have kept at it for my dog."

Dogs Elevate Exercise from Drudgery to Joyful Routine

JANICE Willard, a writer, producer, and veterinarian who lives in Moscow, Idaho, started a rigorous exercise routine with her dogs—not because she was in the mood to get fit, but because a massive winter storm closed the rural road where she lives, and she had to hike to and from her car if she wanted to go anywhere. Actually, she had to do it even if she didn't care to go out, because she had to get her kids to school.

"I was not happy about that development," Dr. Willard says wryly. "In fact, I was miserable. I'm overweight, I have arthritis in my left leg, and the temperatures were in the single digits."

On her first morning trudging down to the car, though, Dr. Willard found that her three dogs, particularly Rosie, an Australian shepherd/golden retriever/little bit of mystery mix, were delighted with the adventure. "The minute I walked out the door, there was Rosie, with her tail flying, jumping through the snowdrifts, running full out, absolutely joyful," says Dr. Willard. "She'd run down to the car and back to me two or three times while I was slogging along, trying to get there once, and she was so happy—to be with me, to be outside, to be playing in the snow. I really did try to stay grumpy, but I didn't have a chance. Rosie's enthusiasm was infectious."

Since that fateful snowstorm, Dr. Willard has kept up a regular routine of walking with her dogs, more for the euphoria that comes with working out with them than for any other reason—even weight loss. "Whether you walk enough to lose a pound or ten pounds or more, the walking itself is invigorating and uplifting—and it is even more so with an enthusiastic dog," she observes.

A Well-Exercised Dog Is a Good Dog

THE fringe benefit of a workout program that includes your dog is a big one: as any experienced trainer can tell you, a well-exercised, tired dog is a well-behaved dog, too. Common canine behavior problems such as biting, barking, digging, chewing, house soiling (a problem which, by way of euthanasia, is the number one cause of death in dogs in the United States and results in more deaths than accidents, cancer, and infectious disease combined) have a wonderful way of disappearing when the dog in question is getting enough exercise every day. A panting dog not only looks and feels better, he often gets a new "leash on life" as the regime exercises both the body and the mind.

Sandi Martin, a nurse from Salt Lake City, Utah, is an expert in human health and dog behavior. She founded a program that uses therapy dogs to help children overcome reading difficulties. Sandi's Portuguese water dog, Zelda, sits quietly on kids' laps, gazing intently at the pages of a book while each child reads aloud. From time to time, Zelda taps her paw to the rhythm of the syllables to help the reader sound out a word. Her nonjudgmental, endless patience in her work does not come naturally—the breed requires plenty of physical exercise to achieve that kind of well-mannered ease. The secret, Sandi explains, is two walks a day, one in the morning and one at night. Even though her own idea of a good workout is "a really rugged game of Scrabble," Sandi was willing to get out and walk—often and in all weather—when she got her puppy. "I knew it was part of the commitment of being a pet owner," she says.

THE SNOOZE FACTOR

The Mayo Clinic Sleep Disorder Unit has reported that the number-one reason people have trouble sleeping is (drum roll, please . . .) because of disturbances caused by their family pets. We're here to make a leap from this statistic to this sad fact: Overweight dogs snore! Some snore just a little, and some snore nearly loud enough to wake the dead. If improving your dog's behavior isn't enough to motivate you to stick with the Fitness Unleashed routine, how about the prospect of a long, restful, snore-free night's sleep next to your newly lean dog instead?

Sandi knew holding up her end of that commitment would make Zelda easier to train and manage as a therapy dog, but she wasn't prepared for the unexpected bonus of her new routine: over the course of six months, with little or no change in her lifestyle except her twice-daily walks with Zelda, Sandi lost twenty-four pounds.

She confides that as much as she loves Zelda, and as well trained as the little powerhouse of a dog is, Sandi knows if she ever tried to slip back into couch-potato mode, it's unlikely there'd be any couch left to sit on. "Zelda would demolish it while I was at work," Sandi laughs. "She really does need her exercise."

Dogs Help You Appreciate Nature and the Neighborhood

DOUG WHITTAKER has lived in the Catskill mountains in upstate New York all his life. He lives out in the country, with acres of woods, hills, clearings, and natural beauty. He'll be the first to tell

THE VETERINARIAN SAYS

One of the things I love most about walking with our golden retriever, Shakira, is how our adventures make me feel connected with nature. What I experience on my daily walks ranges from average (a deer) to awesome (a herd of elk) to out-of-this-world (a momma bear and her two cubs ten feet away . . . yikes!). I live in the mountains of the Idaho Panhandle, near the Canadian border, and it seems Mother Nature played favorites here. Hundreds of species of animals call our ranch home. On our daily walks, Shakira and I have seen moose, elk, bears, a cougar, coyotes, and dozens of birds and small animals ranging from bald eagles and giant woodpeckers to squirrels, snowshoe rabbits, and ermine.

We've discovered old dumps where homesteaders tossed their trash and we've retrieved bottles now purple with sun-ripened age, and we've found a tree where lovers had carved their commitment into the bark, never expecting a scampering squirrel to point it out to us as he raced up the trunk.

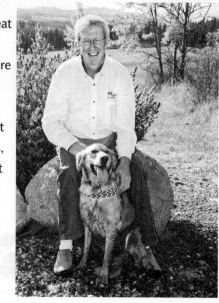

Perhaps better than the sweat and sensory treats we encounter on our daily walks are the times afterwards when I sit on a log and pet Shakira and relish a moment without deadlines, electronic tethers, or artificial stimulations. Just silence and peace.

THE DOCTOR SAYS

As an avid jogger, I'm used to running through our neighborhood, clearing my mind of the day's tasks but never really taking the time to stop and smell the roses. Walking our Havanese puppy, Cooper, has changed all that. This adorable, smiling, black-and-white-spotted pup hops like a bunny and is a people magnet. Everyone stops, stares, and smiles—and most ask what kind of dog Cooper is (most people have never heard of a Ha-

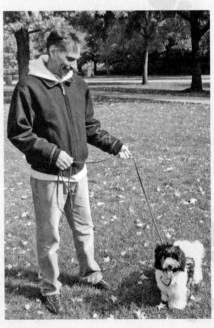

vanese). My wife, Nancy, always says with a smile: "Your next dog!"

In addition to helping Nancy and me catch up with our neighbors and meet new people, our walks with Cooper also sensitize us to our neighborhood's sights, sounds, and smells. Birds chirping, children skateboarding, a squirrel running up a tree, the buzz of an airplane flying overhead, or an ambulance siren may seem mundane in the land of suburbia, but not when experiencing them for the first time through Cooper's curious eyes and ears!

When I choose to go out jogging (which I still enjoy), it's just another part of my routine. Each and every time I pick up the leash to walk Cooper, though, he looks at me, wriggling and wagging his tail as if I'm about to take him to Disney World for the first time. It would have been much cheaper and easier raising our children if such simple neighborhood outings had elicited a similar response!

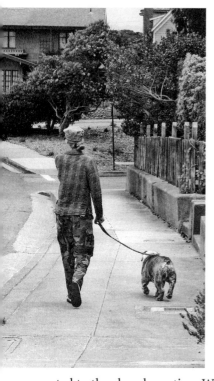

you that he really gets to appreciate his land and its natural splendors most during his daily walks with his dogs. Doug and his wife, Cynthia, have a Lab and two corgis and walk them at least a mile, and often much more, on uneven, steep terrain each day. The couple attributes their fitness to the time they spend outdoors, and neither could imagine taking on any other exercise regimen.

"We've had a few pieces of fitness equipment in the house over the years," Doug says. "We had an exercise bike, a treadmill, and weights. Some of it's in the storeroom now, and some of it we donated to the church auction. We never used it much."

One of the greatest pleasures of walking a dog is getting out in the world, seeing people, feeling the weather and the fresh air. For those who live in rural areas, it's an opportunity to appreciate nature. If you live in town, the benefits of walking your dog are no less. While the opportunities to enjoy the sun and the sky and the breeze are still there, getting out for a walk can be fulfilling for those who like to keep to themselves and also for those who love to make new friends. Sandi Martin explains that one of the reasons she has come to enjoy Zelda's walks almost as much as the dog does is simply that she's a "people person." "We get out and meet people and wave hello to the neighbors and really explore our route," Sandi says. "I love getting to know the city this way."

SUNSHINE ON YOUR SHOULDERS

Recent studies from around the world have shown the role of Vitamin D (the sunshine vitamin) in health is far more important and complex than just as a necessary ingredient for strong bones. Vitamin D is proving to preserve muscle strength and to give people some protection against deadly diseases including multiple sclerosis, diabetes, and even cancer. What better way to get your daily dose than getting out and walking your dog?

Dogs Take the Focus off You

UNDERTAKING a walking or jogging routine alone can make anyone feel excruciatingly self-conscious. With every step, you may feel like bystanders are thinking, "It's about time." Walk or jog with a dog, however, and suddenly you are a doer of good deeds, an animal lover, a good sport who doesn't mind being dragged around the block a few times by an eager pet. The difference may be in your head, but studies show most people do feel more comfortable walking with a dog than without one.

"There are not a lot of socially acceptable ways for fat people to exercise," says Janice Willard. Whether or not they're significantly overweight, many people relish having a "reason" to walk. With a pet at your side, it really doesn't matter how you look, or how you're dressed. People automatically attach positive social attributes to you (i.e., she must be a good person) and are attracted by your combined gravitational pull.

DOGS ON LOAN: FINDING A DOG TO WALK— WHEN YOU DON'T HAVE ONE OF YOUR OWN

So, no dog? That doesn't mean you can't walk one. If you or someone you know would like to walk someone else's dog, here are three ways to find one:

Visit the animal shelter—Shelter staff are notoriously overworked and underpaid (they're often not paid at all). Though they would love to be able to walk all the dogs in their care, many simply do not have the resources to make this happen. If you'd like to combine your workout with a very good deed, check in at your local shelter to see if you can walk dogs for them on a regular schedule. Chances are, both the staff and the dogs will be happy to have you. In fact, some shelters, including facilities in Lubbock, Texas; Indianapolis, Indiana; and Reno, Nevada, participate in a program called Walk a Pound, Lose a Pound, which pairs for outings good Samaritans looking for a brisk walk and dogs desperately needing the exercise.

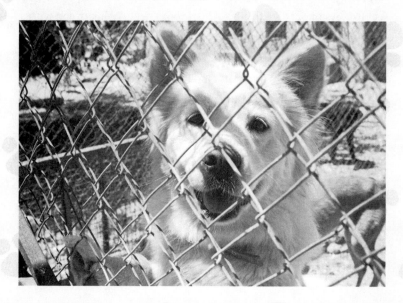

Look around the neighborhood—We know of far too many homes where people have dogs but not the time, energy, or physical ability to provide the exercise they need. If you know someone who is elderly, families with small children, single parents, or a friend who works long hours and leaves a dog at home, consider offering to walk the dog. You don't have to make a long-term commitment—suggest that you'd like to try out dog walking for exercise (or maybe as a prelude to getting a dog of your own) and wondered if you and the family's dog could help each other.

Inquire at a boarding kennel or veterinary hospital—If only kennel staff would walk our dogs more, we might leave them there more often. A boarding kennel has everything to gain by ensuring that its dogs get plenty of exercise (see page 44, "A Well-Exercised Dog Is a Good Dog"). If you play your cards right when you have this discussion with a kennel owner, you might even get paid for dog walking. Kennels often charge extra for each walk given to dogs over the course of their stay. Veterinary hospitals often offer "play times" for animals that are boarded, too.

Consider this research on this topic: A British study followed a woman with a yellow Lab as she went about her daily routine for five days, and then for five days without the dog. With the dog, she spoke with 156 people. Without the dog, she interacted with 50. Researcher June McNicholas, a professor of psychology at the University of Warwick, pointed to the interactions stimulated by the dog as the key to a better sense of psychological well-being. The positive attention and goodwill that strangers extended to the dog toggled up the leash to the woman at the end of it, too.

It's a Good Deed

CREATIVE and compassionate, Rebecca Johnson, professor of nursing and veterinary medicine at the University of Missouri at Columbia, decided the health benefits of dog ownership shouldn't be confined to people who own dogs; so she designed a program to share the wealth. When she launched her Walking for Healthy Hearts program at the university, Dr. Johnson created walking partnerships by pairing certified therapy dogs with a group of economically disadvantaged, disabled adults from a housing development. The initial goal of the program was simply to get the participants out of the house, encourage them to get some exercise, and see what health benefits might develop. Dr. Johnson had high hopes for her program, but it was an entirely new method, and she was going to have to just wait and see.

At the start of the program, Dr. Johnson had participants walk ten minutes per day, three times each week. Over the course of several weeks, sessions were increased to thirty minutes per day, five days a week. Each walker was given a full health assessment at the beginning of the study, measuring weight, lean body mass, bone density, blood pressure, blood sugar, cholesterol, triglycerides, and joint movement functional ability.

What happened over the course of that first year was both remarkable and magical. The participants in the study, every one suffering from some chronic illness or physical or mental impairment, a group that was almost entirely sedentary at the outset of the program, embraced walking with the study dogs as if they'd been waiting for the opportunity all their lives. "People have been absolutely devoted to this program," says Dr. Johnson. "They've said things like, 'The dogs make me a better person,' and 'Now I have a reason to get up in the morning.' We actually have one participant who started this program in a motorized wheelchair and ended it walking around the block on his feet." One participant reported, choked up but smiling, "I never thought I could feel this good again."

The participants didn't sign on to the program for the purpose of weight loss, and they were not given any nutrition-related advice, but the walkers lost an average of 14.4 pounds. Some lost more than 30. In addition, they rated themselves as being less depressed and more physically fit at the end of the study than at its beginning.

The dedication and success of this exercise program boils down to one thing, says Dr. Johnson: the presence of the dogs, and the dedication they inspired in the participants. Time and again, Dr. Johnson was told by walkers that they had come, despite a physical ailment or inclement weather or depression, because they knew the dogs needed them, would miss them, or would miss out on the walk.

In exit interviews for the People and Pets Exercising Together study, Dr. Kushner received similar feedback from his participants. One reported, "If it weren't for my dog, I would not go out on daily walks." Another wrote, "Caring for and loving my dog is what motivated me to be a part of this program." A third said, "Knowing I could do something good for my dog was my motivating factor."

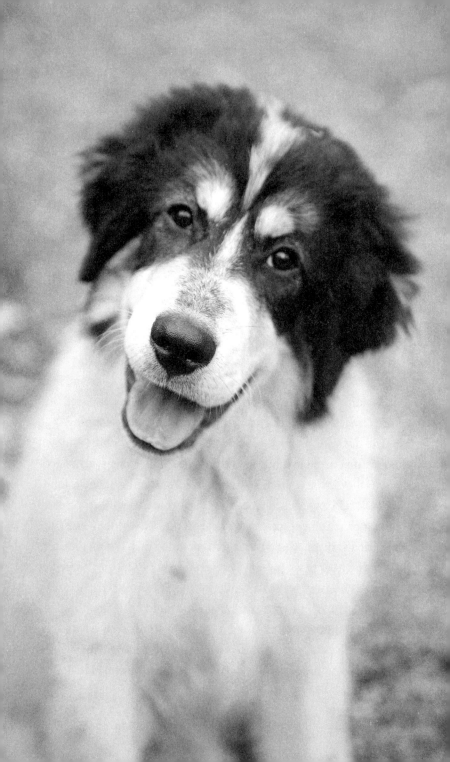

PART II

A
Plan of
Action

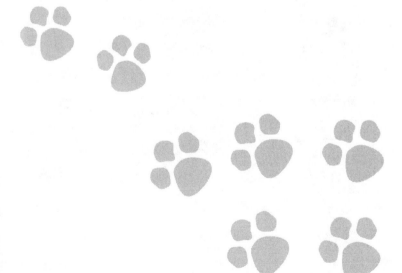

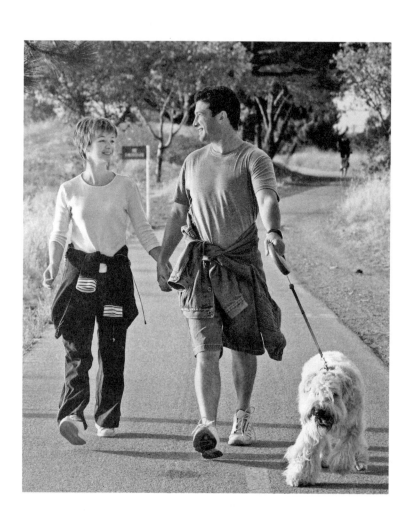

CHAPTER 3

People Patterns:
Pinpointing Your Personal
Eating and Exercise Habits

Over the years, Jane Rudnitsky of Oneonta, New York, has been on a cabbage-soup diet, a low-fat diet, a no-carb diet, and even a crazy seven-food/seven-day diet ("Seven bananas on one day, seven hot dogs on another," she explains. "Don't ask me why—I was young and foolish then.") In addition, the forty-year-old mother of two teenagers has tried aqua aerobics, Pilates, stationary biking, tae-bo, and yoga, among other activities, to increase her activity level and lose weight. Some of the exercise regimens and diets yielded results, but nothing lasted. Every time a program petered out because the diet was too restrictive or the class or exercise routine wasn't her cup of tea, Jane started at square one again, with the same feelings of being tired and overweight and out of ideas for tackling the problem.

While Jane was at most of her fitness classes, her chocolate Labrador retriever, Zeke, was home in a crate, getting bigger and wilder with every passing week. "I'd want to walk him around the block when I got home, and he'd pull at the leash and act like a crazy dog," she explains. "It made it hard to walk him at all."

It wasn't until she and her dog started getting their exercise together that Jane's fitness regimen finally "clicked" and she realized she'd found something she could stick to for the long term. She started by walking Zeke for a few blocks in the spring. Jane enjoyed the invigorating feeling of getting outside and getting moving, and worked up to a two-mile loop, then even farther. These days, Jane and Zeke take what she calls their "detox walk"—a challenging six-mile route that canvasses their small town—at least a couple of times a week in addition to shorter jaunts.

While she still sometimes attends a class or pops in an exercise tape, Jane is positive that walking the dog is the fitness solution she's spent much of her adult life looking for. Over a full year of long walks, she's lost 30 pounds and dropped three sizes. As the weight came off, she gained a sense of strength and control over her body— a feeling that extended to making smarter dietary choices, too. "I take smaller portions and eat less junk," she says. "Once I was feeling better about myself, it wasn't nearly as hard as it used to be to control my eating."

Why did dog walking work when tae-bo and aqua aerobics did not? For starters, Jane says, walking qualifies as hard-to-find "me" time. "I guess you could say it's like working out and relaxing at the same time," she explains. Going to the gym felt like a chore, but after being at work all day, she loves the solitude and her easy companionship with Zeke. Even though she pushes herself to walk far and fast, and to work her way through hilly terrain, Jane enjoys the fresh air, the views, and the physical effort. It's even better when her children decide to join her, she says, because with no video games, no television, and no ringing phone, she gets to hear about everything that's going on in their lives as they walk. As for Zeke, "He's a different dog.

He's so cool now. Nothing bothers him as long as he gets enough exercise. He literally lives for the moment when I get the leash out."

No One-Size Solution

FINDING an exercise and diet solution you can live with—not just for a few days or weeks, but indefinitely—is the key to successfully losing weight and gaining health. Like Jane, most of us try a number of different methods before figuring out what works. Some of those methods are ridiculous (like a food-of-the-day diet, juice-only diet, or a milk-shake diet), and others are poor fits for our preferences and lifestyles (like an aerobics class for a person who feels clumsy and self-conscious even when standing still, or an early-morning hour at the gym for a night owl with a full-time job and a child to get ready for school). At the Wellness Institute at Northwestern Memorial Hospital in Chicago, where Dr. Kushner is the medical director, pinpointing each patient's existing diet and exercise patterns through quizzes and interviews is the first step in any treatment. The benefits of taking the time to get to know the patients are twofold: First, going through this process helps both the institute's staff and the patient understand what kinds of habits and lifestyle factors contributed to the extra weight in the first place. Second, with that understanding in place, the treatment team and the patient can work together to find a treatment plan that's realistic and effective.

Peggy Mitchell, a clinical exercise physiologist and manager of the institute, welcomes newcomers with an interview about their backgrounds, likes, dislikes, and habits. After reviewing each client's health history, she quizzes them about what kinds of activities or sports they enjoyed as a child, in school, and as an adult, how they spend their leisure time, and what their average day is like. She asks

THE DOCTOR SAYS

When we talk about diet plans for weight loss, it's often in terms of carbs, grams of protein, fat intake, and calories burned. While those factors can all contribute to the success or failure of a program, my research identifies three entirely different issues as more significant: the habits of procrastinating, people pleasing, and setting unrealistic goals.

The problem with following any diet plan is that life "gets in the way." Stress, illness, obstacles, priorities, and other responsibilities often trump our best intentions to lose weight. For example, the procrastinator puts off making the necessary changes, people pleasers consistently prioritize the needs of others above their own, and overreaching achievers set the bar so high that no progress or improvement is good enough—and they soon give up because their goals seem impossible to meet. One of the great, surprising benefits of establishing an exercise program with your dog is that it subtly addresses these common roadblocks to weight loss. For people pleasers, such as parents juggling the obligations of their children and trying to balance professional priorities, too, taking care of others is second nature. But sticking to a dog-walking program *does* address a significant need on the part of another family member—the dog. I've found that many patients are willing to stick to the program for their dogs, even when they would otherwise feel guilty about setting aside time for exercise.

A canine companion is an ideal partner for procrastinators, too. While walking buddies may come and go—or be easy to cancel with a phone call or an e-mail—dogs can be remarkably insistent on getting their scheduled walks. There's nothing quite like the immediacy of an edgy, eager, unrelenting dog to remind a procrastinator that there's no time like the present. For dogs, "now" doesn't mean fifteen minutes later.

Lastly, in the case of overachievers, walking with a dog creates a built-in short-term goal—to make your dog happy, tired, and well behaved one day at a time.

I never expected, when I started studying ways to help people lose weight and take better care of themselves, that I'd find such an effective ally in the average canine companion. If the research continues to demonstrate what terrific weight-loss "tools" dogs are, the time may come when we medical professionals recommend to our patients to get puppies as often as we do to drink lots of water, eat fruits and vegetables, and get enough sleep at night.

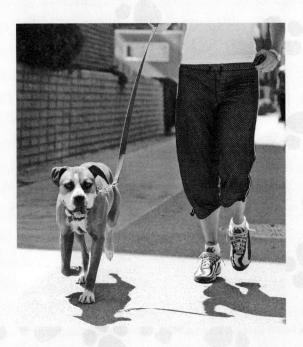

clients how they feel about exercise, and about the kinds of food choices they usually make. The exercise questions help Peggy figure out what kinds of activities might suit each person. As she explains, "If I find that someone is very social, and I recommend forty-five minutes a day riding a stationary bike in front of the television, I'm wasting her time. I try to help each client find activities that will have some intrinsic appeal—some kind of a 'hook' that will hold their interest and get them going. It's got to be something that's a match for the patient's personality."

Dogs, it turns out, are a wonderful hook. It wasn't until she saw the enthusiasm and success of the People and Pets Exercising Together participants (who met at the Wellness Institute during the study) that Peggy realized she might be overlooking a few important questions in her interviews. "Now, I always ask if the client has a dog; what kind of dog it is; how much exercise it gets; and if, when, and where the dog is already being walked," she explains. "By incorporating dogs in an exercise plan, we find that the people we treat are more willing to follow through with their programs."

Figuring Out Where You Fit In

THINK about a cross-section of adults who are overweight or obese: a twenty-six-year-old stay-at-home mom who snacks all day and doesn't get enough sleep at night; a forty-five-year-old executive who eats all her meals in the car and in restaurants; a fifty-three-year-old teacher who watches TV and snacks at night when he's feeling bored; a person from a "foodie" family who doesn't know the first thing about portion control. Giving all of these people identical instructions for getting into shape—with cookie-cutter diet plans and blanket instructions for working out—would be a long shot at best.

THE DOCTOR SAYS: GREAT GOALS

It's pretty common for me to meet with a patient who loves everything about her life—except her hips. At the Wellness Institute, we help and encourage patients to reach their weight and fitness goals and realize a positive self-image. Sometimes, though, I have to take a minute to bring up the very real differences between the "standard" we see every day in the media and the standards I believe in and uphold as a health professional. The average female model is five feet ten inches tall and weighs about 120 pounds. She may look great in pictures, but she is significantly underweight. In fact, any weight between 132 and 170 pounds is healthy for that height. For your reference, we've included a BMI chart at the back of the book. Keep in mind that if you are very muscular, you may be at, or even over, the top weight for your height and still be in excellent condition.

The right way to embark upon the Fitness Unleashed program is to assess your personal eating and exercise habits. For this dog owner–oriented book, we've customized the exercise portion of the test for people with dogs at home. Are you a Meal Skipper? A Steady Snacker? Are you the Doggie Doorkeeper? Or maybe a Stop-and-Go Stroller? Take the following Fitness Unleashed Personality Quiz and review the results. Once you find your categories (and your dog's, in the next chapter!), we'll help you customize a plan to address your unique strengths and weaknesses so that you can lose weight and gain health.

The Fitness Unleashed Personality Quiz

Check the answer that best reflects your level of agreement with each statement.

Part I: What Kind of Eater Are You?

1. I eat when the mood strikes me, or when hunger dictates, but not on any particular schedule.
   a. Not me at all. (0 pts)
   b. This is true quite often. (1 pt)
   c. This is me most of the time. (2 pts)
   d. That's me. (3 pts)

2. When I see or smell foods I like, I feel I have to take a bite, or two, or more.
   a. Not me at all. (0 pts)
   b. This is true quite often. (1 pt)
   c. This is me most of the time. (2 pts)
   d. That's me. (3 pts)

3. I don't give much thought to portion sizes. I more or less fill my plate.
   a. Not me at all. (0 pts)
   b. This is true quite often. (1 pt)
   c. This is me most of the time. (2 pts)
   d. That's me. (3 pts)

4. I have a hard time passing through the kitchen at home or at work without picking up something extra to snack on.
   a. Not me at all. (0 pts)
   b. This is true quite often. (1 pt)

c. This is me most of the time. (2 pts)

d. That's me. (3 pts)

5. I skip meals, especially early in the day.

    a. Not me at all. (0 pts)

    b. This is true quite often. (1 pt)

    c. This is me most of the time. (2 pts)

    d. That's me. (3 pts)

6. I snack a lot, even when I'm not hungry.

    a. Not me at all. (0 pts)

    b. This is true quite often. (1 pt)

    c. This is me most of the time. (2 pts)

    d. That's me. (3 pts)

7. I eat fast and before I know it, I've eaten more than I meant to—sometimes so much I feel uncomfortably full.

    a. Not me at all. (0 pts)

    b. This is true quite often. (1 pt)

    c. This is me most of the time. (2 pts)

    d. That's me. (3 pts)

8. If I don't choose the healthiest food option, I feel really guilty.

    a. Not me at all. (0 pts)

    b. This is true quite often. (1 pt)

    c. This is me most of the time. (2 pts)

    d. That's me. (3 pts)

9. I rarely plan my meals.

    a. Not me at all. (0 pts)

    b. This is true quite often. (1 pt)

    c. This is me most of the time. (2 pts)

    d. That's me. (3 pts)

10. I eat "good" foods when I'm around others, but when I'm alone I let myself eat the "bad" foods.
    a. Not me at all. (0 pts)
    b. This is true quite often. (1 pt)
    c. This is me most of the time. (2 pts)
    d. That's me. (3 pts)

11. It's common for me to leave the table feeling stuffed.
    a. Not me at all. (0 pts)
    b. This is true quite often. (1 pt)
    c. This is me most of the time. (2 pts)
    d. That's me. (3 pts)

12. I battle between what I want to eat and what I think I should eat, which never leaves me feeling satisfied.
    a. Not me at all. (0 pts)
    b. This is true quite often. (1 pt)
    c. This is me most of the time. (2 pts)
    d. That's me. (3 pts)

Here's How to Score Your Eating Habits

Add points from questions 1, 5, and 9 to get your
MEAL SKIPPER score: _____

Add points from questions 2, 4, and 6 to get your
STEADY SNACKER score: _____

Add points from questions 3, 7, and 11 to get your
HEARTY PORTIONER score: _____

Add points from questions 8, 10, and 12 to get your
SWING EATER score: _____

The highest total score reveals your dominant eating-personality type. If there's a tie among your highest scores, then pick the one eating pattern that you most relate to. See pattern descriptions below.

Eating Personalities

MEAL SKIPPER

You skip meals and have no structure to your eating patterns. Eating is an afterthought, occurring anytime or anywhere. When the day is done, you don't have a clue as to what or how much you ate. This cycle of unplanned eating gets repeated day after day.

Three steps to start making your eating personality more healthful:

● Pinky-swear you'll eat three meals a day—breakfast, lunch, and dinner. We're willing to bet your caloric intake is dropping and spiking on your irregular eating schedule. Your body needs regular, dependable meals to function at its most effective level, and in order for you to learn to listen to your internal cues for hunger and fullness, you can't wait until you're famished before you think about your next meal.

● Concentrate—on your meals. When you eat, please focus your attention on the dining experience. If you're also driving, watching TV, surfing the Internet, or running to a meeting, you're not going to be fully satisfied with your food, and you're not going to be in tune with those fullness cues we were just talking about.

● Drink more water. If the reason you're skipping meals is because you're on the run, odds are you're not taking the time to drink enough water, either. By the time you're really, really hungry and ready to overindulge, you're also bordering on dehydration. Drinking water regularly through the day will help you control your hunger, and it will help remind you that you need to nourish your body.

STEADY SNACKER

You start out committed to eating three meals a day, but a lot of unplanned snacking is going on throughout the day—even when you're not really hungry. Some Steady Snackers eat because they're bored, and some snack because the sight or smell of food can trigger the compulsion to eat. Since we live in a culture where we are seeing and smelling food everywhere, the snacking quickly adds up to excess calories and weight gain.

Three steps to start making your eating personality more healthful:

- Write it down. Yes, keeping a food diary is pretty inconvenient for a Steady Snacker—it probably means taking notes all day long. For many people who fall into this category, seeing exactly how much food they've taken in over the course of a day—and figuring out how many calories it adds up to—is a sobering experience that can help change their habits for the better.
- Clean the cupboards. One of the characteristics of this eating personality is that you find it hard to resist snacking on foods wherever you find them. You may not be able to control all the food triggers in the workplace, the mall, or even on the side of the road, but you can limit the kind and quantity of goodies in your own home.
- Take one planned treat—or two. There's nothing wrong with snacking—as long as you're not doing it all day long. Pick one or two favorite items each day, measure out the portion you intend to eat, and enjoy it. Then don't go back for more. This is very hard in the beginning, but if you can stick to it for just a week, you'll find it does get easier.

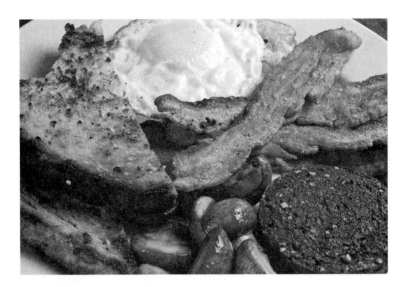

HEARTY PORTIONER

Hearty Portioners put too much food on their plates, usually finish it, and feel stuffed. You eat quickly and really aren't sure what constitutes a normal, healthy portion of any food. You're a frequent member of the clean-plate club, but you'd rather be able to enjoy your meals without overeating.

Three steps to start making your eating personality more healthful:

● Read labels (and count and measure portions) for one week. Count the crackers. Measure the cereal. Weigh the meat. Just a few days of taking a close look at what qualifies as one serving will be an eye-opener for any Hearty Portioner.

● Stop and breathe. Five minutes into your meal, put down your fork, swallow what's in your mouth, and stop eating for a full minute. Do you feel full? If not, repeat in five minutes.

● Pick a new plate. Use a smaller plate, or rearrange your old one. Choose meat portions the size of a deck of cards and starch portions equal to 1 cup. Fill up the rest of your plate with fruits and vegetables.

SWING EATER

Swing Eaters eat "good" foods in public and "bad" foods in private and never feel satisfied. You have an internal battle going on between what you think you should be eating and what you like to eat. You swing from severely restricting your eating to overindulging. You'd like to achieve a healthier eating style but you're not sure how to do it.

Three steps to start making your eating personality more healthful:

- Love your food. All of it. The first thing a Swing Eater needs to accept is that there are no forbidden foods and that there's nothing constructive about pairing eating and feelings of shame. Make a conscious decision to choose moderate portions of foods you enjoy at mealtimes, and also a conscious decision to start cutting back on those foods between meals.

- Fill up. Incorporating fiber, healthy fats, and even sweets in your daily diet will help you overcome the impulse to divide foods into the categories of good and evil. It's okay to cook with healthy fats like olive oil, and it's okay to have small dessert servings. Choose a preportioned treat to enjoy once a day—such as a 100-calorie fudge Popsicle or a 100-calorie package of your favorite crackers—so you don't feel deprived.

- Don't hide. The bag of M&Ms at the back of the cupboard has to go, as does the stash of chips in the trunk. You can have these foods in small portions, but you need to learn to eat them in public and in front of your family so you can start having a more healthy relationship with food in general.

Good Advice for Every Eating Personality

In addition to the previous customized advice, here are three suggestions that will benefit any weight-loss program. These recommendations have proven helpful in the successful treatment of thousands of patients at the Wellness Institute. They are suitable for every eating type, and also for eaters who feel they're doing "all the right stuff" and are just looking for an extra bit of nutrition wisdom.

● Eat more fruits and vegetables. Eating more of anything runs counter to most people's understanding of "diet," but over the long haul, most successful weight-loss programs help participants increase their intake of high-fiber, nutrient-rich fruits and vegetables and reduce their intake of starches and sweets. Although many recently popular diet programs advise against consuming some kinds of fruits and vegetables because of their high carbohydrate content, in *Fitness Unleashed* we don't recommend any such restrictions. It's simply important to remember that all foods—even the ones that are good for your body—do have calories and so need to be consumed in moderate portions.

At the Wellness Institute, it's recommended that patients try to add a fruit or vegetable to every meal and try to eat them for between-meal snacks as well. Many of the patients have had great success in taking this advice to heart when cooking. In any recipe for a casserole, stir-fry, or pasta combination, for example, try reducing the quantity of meat by a third and doubling the amount of vegetables.

● Practice portion control. For many of our patients, relying on preportioned meals and snacks or meal-replacement bars in the early days of their weight-loss programs is a tremendous help in the long run. We don't recommend that you spend the rest of your days eating nothing but frozen dinners or individually packaged snacks, but eating products such as Lean Cuisine or Healthy Choice frozen meals for a week or two can help you get a feel for what a "real" single portion looks like. You may occasionally want to stock a few in the freezer for times when you want an easy meal you know isn't overly high in calories and fat. Meal-replacement bars like Kashi Go Lean, Balance, or Clif can make quick meals on the run. Feel free to supplement these kinds of meals and snacks with a portion of a fresh vegetable or fruit.

Enlist your friends and family. We know your dog is going to back you up in the exercise department, but if you live in a home or spend a lot of time in an environment where everyone else is indulging in junk food and huge portions, it's an extreme challenge to stick to your plan all by yourself. Tell the people you love and trust that you've made a decision to eat healthier, and ask them to help you by offering their support and encouragement. Many of the Wellness Institute's patients are the primary shoppers and food preparers for their families. Inevitably, it's an adjustment for the whole family when the person who performs those functions chooses to change his or her eating habits. Over the years, though, the Institute's health providers have had hundreds of patients come back and thank them for their sound nutritional advice and tell them that their entire families adjusted and benefited from the changes they implemented at home.

Part II: What's Your Dog-Walking Profile?

1. My dog and I go in and out the door together so he can do his business in the yard. That's about as far as we usually get.
   a. Not me at all. (0 pts)
   b. This is true quite often. (1 pt)
   c. This is me most of the time. (2 pts)
   d. That's me. (3 pts)

2. Walking my dog involves more stopping and going than huffing and puffing.
   a. Not me at all. (0 pts)
   b. This is true quite often. (1 pt)
   c. This is me most of the time. (2 pts)
   d. That's me. (3 pts)

3. My dog and I have been taking long walks on the same favorite route for years.
   a. Not me at all. (0 pts)
   b. This is true quite often. (1 pt)
   c. This is me most of the time. (2 pts)
   d. That's me. (3 pts)

4. I don't walk my dog if it's hot, cold, or if there's precipitation.
   a. Not me at all. (0 pts)
   b. This is true quite often. (1 pt)
   c. This is me most of the time. (2 pts)
   d. That's me. (3 pts)

5. I consistently walk my dog at least four days a week for thirty minutes or more.
   a. Not me at all. (0 pts)
   b. This is true quite often. (1 pt)
   c. This is me most of the time. (2 pts)
   d. That's me. (3 pts)

6. I get a good workout at the gym, then take my dog around the block when I get home.
   a. Not me at all. (0 pts)
   b. This is true quite often. (1 pt)
   c. This is me most of the time. (2 pts)
   d. That's me. (3 pts)

7. I'm almost never tired, winded, or sweaty after a walk with my dog.
   a. Not me at all. (0 pts)
   b. This is true quite often. (1 pt)
   c. This is me most of the time. (2 pts)
   d. That's me. (3 pts)

8. My dog and I spend a lot of time together on the couch.
   a. Not me at all. (0 pts)
   b. This is true quite often. (1 pt)
   c. This is me most of the time. (2 pts)
   d. That's me. (3 pts)

9. I don't walk my dog much because he's too slow/too old/sniffs too much/too busy making pit stops to keep up with my vigorous pace.
   a. Not me at all. (0 pts)
   b. This is true quite often. (1 pt)
   c. This is me most of the time. (2 pts)
   d. That's me. (3 pts)

10. I walk my dog at a steady pace, and I usually break a sweat.
    a. Not me at all. (0 pts)
    b. This is true quite often. (1 pt)
    c. This is me most of the time. (2 pts)
    d. That's me. (3 pts)

11. I get plenty of exercise, but my dog is pretty much a couch potato.
    a. Not me at all. (0 pts)
    b. This is true quite often. (1 pt)
    c. This is me most of the time. (2 pts)
    d. That's me. (3 pts)

12. My dog and I walk at a leisurely pace, which leaves plenty of time for his sniffing and exploring.
    a. Not me at all. (0 pts)
    b. This is true quite often. (1 pt)
    c. This is me most of the time. (2 pts)
    d. That's me. (3 pts)

Here's How to Score Your Dog-Walking Profile

Are you getting the most from your time with your dog? Is your dog getting "full benefits" from you? Follow these directions to find out:

Add points from questions 1, 4, and 8 to get your
DOGGIE DOORKEEPER score: _____

Add points from questions 2, 7, and 12 to get your
STOP-AND-GO STROLLER score: _____

Add points from questions 3, 5, and 10 to get your
SAME-ROUTE REPEATER score: _____

Add points from questions 6, 9, and 11 to get your
FUR-FREE FITNESS FAN score: _____

The highest total score reveals your dominant dog-walking personality type. If there's a tie among your highest scores, then pick the pattern that you most relate to. See pattern descriptions below.

Exercise Personalities

DOGGIE DOORKEEPER

Cue music from that overplayed Baha Men hit song: You let the dog out. You let the dog in. End of story. It's an important job, and somebody has to do it. Unfortunately, all the getting up and getting down and opening and closing of doors doesn't add up to much of a physical effort for you or your pooch. You may get extra points for taking out the garbage on the way or bending over to pick up the newspaper, and your dog may score a few for chasing the occasional squirrel in the yard, but now's a great time to plan some significant movement for both of you. In Chapter 6, we'll explain why your sedentary lifestyle may actually make it easier for you to start losing weight, and we'll help you get started on the right foot.

STOP-AND-GO STROLLER

Any exercise is better than none at all, so for starters, pat yourself on the back for the effort you're making to get up, get moving, and take good care of your own body and your dog's health. That said, if you want dog walking to help you take off extra pounds (and it can!), we're going to help you revamp your routine to make it more consistent (even on bad-weather days, days when you're extra-busy, or days when you're feeling aches and pains) and more challenging. In Chapter 6, we'll give you a customized program to get your dog walks working harder for you.

SAME-ROUTE REPEATER

You walk; you huff and puff; you sweat. But you're not getting any results. Falling into an exercise rut with your dog-walking routine is an all-too-common problem and one that can be remedied. You probably walk your dog on a lengthy trek at least three times a week, and maybe every day, but your body isn't challenged by your routine and you need to make it longer or more intense to get results. In Chapter 6, we'll give you a detailed, proven plan for taking the workout you've become accustomed to and translating it into one that'll help your body start burning fat and losing weight.

FUR-FREE FITNESS FAN

You're already working out. Good for you! But you have a state-of-the-art, supereffective exercise tool in your home that's not being put to good use. If your workouts aren't having the full effect you're after—or if your dog is letting you know with bad behavior or poor health that he's not getting enough exercise—it may be time to break out the leash and unleash the fitness potential the two of you have as a team. In Chapter 6, we'll show you how you and your dog can become each other's most effective, reliable workout buddy.

In the next chapter, you'll take eating- and exercise-personality quizzes on behalf of your dog. (Hey, we know he's smart, but not *that* smart. . . .) Then turn to Chapter 6 for workout plans that are perfect for the Doggie Doorkeeper, the Stop-and-Go Stroller, the Same-Route Repeater, and the Fur-Free Fitness Fan.

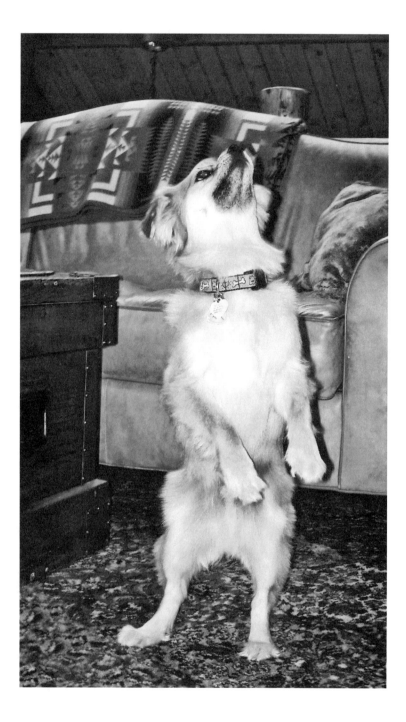

CHAPTER 4

Pet Patterns: Pinpointing Your Dog's Eating and Exercise Habits

When was the last time your dog got up off the couch, ambled into the kitchen, and helped himself to chips or chocolate-chip cookies? Has he skipped breakfast lately to save a couple hundred calories, then gotten so hungry he ate double his normal dinner? Have you ever known him to be wracked with guilt over a weekend of diet indulgences, swearing never to touch cake or cream sauce again?

Not lately? We didn't think so.

For dogs, eating is a much simpler matter than it's become for the tens of millions of people in our society who struggle with weight issues. With few exceptions, dogs are happy to eat whatever you've got, whenever you give it to them, however you give it to them (in their bowl or out of your hand). If they can figure out a way to get more, most will. In addition, they're often content to exercise—or not exercise—as their owners dictate. And if the equation of calories eaten to calories burned adds up to extra pounds, your dog won't give a hoot. Whether you've got a long, lean greyhound or a short, stout

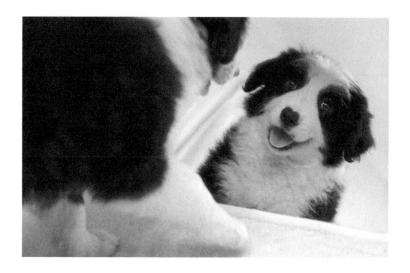

bulldog, he's never going to stop in front of the mirror, look over his shoulder at his furry derrière, and frown or fret and decide it's time to change his life.

As charming as your dog's complete lack of vanity may be, it puts the responsibility for making sure he maintains a healthy weight squarely on you. You may ask yourself why you should bother. You certainly don't love your four-legged best friend any less when he's carrying extra pounds. In fact, in a recent study, the majority of owners of overweight dogs ranked their dogs' weight as "ideal"—the owners weren't even aware the extra pounds were there! It's not as though we weigh Fido after breakfast each morning, and we never have to grouse that he's gained a size and requires a new wardrobe. Unhealthy weight on a dog can be very easy to overlook.

The thing is, though, that the health and longevity benefits for a dog that's kept fit and trim are immense:

- At a healthy weight, your dog will have reduced risk for a host of problems, including cardiac conditions, cancer, osteoarthritis, diabetes, and painful hip and joint ailments.

- At a healthy weight, he'll have more energy and fewer behavioral problems than he would with excess pounds on his frame.
- Most important, research tells us if your dog lives at a healthy weight, his life expectancy is approximately 15 percent longer than if he is overweight or obese. For the average dog, that works out to about two extra years of long walks, tummy rubs, ball chasing, and couch lounging with you.

In this chapter, we'll help you figure out which of your dog's eating and exercise habits (or your own habits in feeding and walking him!) are shaping his long-term health.

Following in Our Footsteps

YEARS ago, America's quintessential dog, Lassie, was out running around the countryside having adventures and trying to save Timmy from peril. But in many modern-day households, you're as likely to find Lassie resting at Timmy's feet while he plays video games as almost anywhere else.

"As we have moved to a more sedentary and pampered culture, so have our pets," explains Dr. Peter Weinstein, medical director of the Veterinary Pet Insurance company. "Today, pets enjoy the same comfort-food choices, plush surroundings, and relaxed lifestyles that many Americans typically enjoy."

Dr. Weinstein should know. In the past three years, his company has seen large increases in the numbers of claims related to heart ailments, diabetes, and joint/back issues—all veterinary conditions frequently linked with being overweight and obese.

Not surprisingly, the state of many pet owners' own health is mirrored by the family dog. Researchers have found that overweight

POUNDS IN PERSPECTIVE

There is no weight/height chart that's effective for figuring out whether a dog is at a healthy weight—except the veterinarian's history of that particular dog's weight over a lifetime. Too much variability exists between (and within) breeds to assign a concrete numeric goal for every dog. If you have a purebred dog, you can refer to the breed standard, but be careful not to put too much stock in this, as your dog may differ from the standard in height and frame—and so have a different ideal weight.

Assessing your dog's weight status means taking a long, hard look at him, explains Tony Buffington, DVM, PhD. For dogs, healthy weight is measured not necessarily in pounds (although the scale at your dog's veterinary office can certainly help), but in body condition. The trick, says Dr. Buffington, is in three assessments:

- A touch of ribs: you shouldn't be able to see your dog's ribs, but you should be able to feel them easily with your fingers. If you have to poke and push through blubber to find the ribs on your dog's sides (like trying to feel the bedsprings through the pillowtop mattress), he probably weighs too much.

- A look at the side: your dog's abdomen should appear tucked up behind the ribs (like a wasp), not hanging down below or bulging alongside.

- The view from the top: when you look down on your dog's back from above, there should be an indentation between the ribs and the hips (like an hourglass). It doesn't have to be a dramatic "waistline," but this is a spot that should curve in, not out.

- In addition to the physical signs of overweight, you can identify it in your dog's health and stamina. If your dog is easily winded, if he has difficulty making the transition from lying down to standing up, or if he's having trouble climbing steps, it may be time to put him on the scale at the veterinarian's office and see if extra weight is slowing him down and taxing his heart, lungs, and frame.

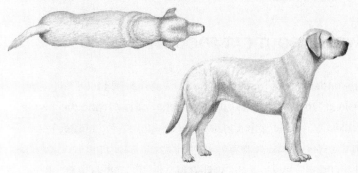

IDEAL

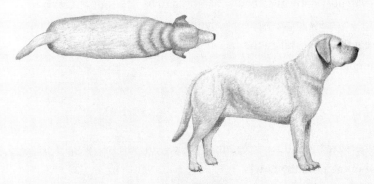

OVERWEIGHT

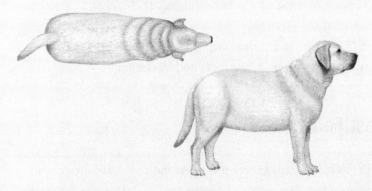

OBESE

A WORD ABOUT CAT-FOOD THIEVES

Ever wonder why so many dogs love to eat the cat's food before the cat can get to it? It's a very common behavior issue, and the answer isn't usually "just to spite the cat"! By design, cat food tastes better than dog food. Cats are notoriously picky eaters, so pet-food companies spend vast budgets and use great scientific minds to create formulas that will entice our feline friends to eat. Dogs aren't nearly as choosy, so even though dog foods are formulated to taste good, they're not nearly as carefully calibrated to be delicious as cat chow. Your dog may be happy to eat anything at all, but he may well choose to eat the good stuff in the cat's bowl first when the opportunity presents itself.

owners are more than three times as likely to own overweight pets as owners at a healthy weight.

"There seems to be a clear link between increasing levels of overweight and obesity in people and increasing incidence of overweight and obesity in dogs," says Tony Buffington, DVM, PhD, a clinical nutritionist at the Ohio State University College of Veterinary Medicine. "We didn't just start noticing this problem that's always been there. Dogs really are getting fatter and less healthy."

Fast Feasts

THE problems dogs experience when they live a low-exercise lifestyle are often compounded by the fact that Mother Nature has equipped them with ferocious, seemingly endless appetites. If you've ever watched your dog polish off a bowl of food in seconds, or worse yet, steal the food of another pet (or person) and all but inhale it, you're familiar with the kind of appetites we're talking about. "Wolfing it down," is the expression that comes to mind, and that's exactly the key to understanding why dogs eat in such a fast and furious way. In the long spectrum of history, they are, after all, not that far evolved from wolves, and even more closely related to generations of self-sufficient dogs who managed to survive on their skills as predators and scavengers. Your pooch may be well groomed and well fed, but his not-so-many-great-grandparents had to catch or find their food—and they had to eat it quickly, or another dog, or some other creature, would.

The instinct to eat as much as possible as fast as possible is still strong in many individual dogs, and also prevalent in many breeds. Labrador retrievers, for example, are notorious in the pet-food and veterinary industries for their willingness to eat anything—and to eat it at record speed. In fact, most pet-food research programs have banned Labs as taste testers because they simply do not discriminate any subtle difference between foods. Beagles, basset hounds, cockers, collies, pugs, and dachshunds are also in this category of anything-goes, swallow-it-whole eaters.

The minimal number of taste buds your dog has further contributes to his strong drive to fill up on any available food. While the average person has about 10,000 taste buds, the average dog has just 1,500. That may help explain why so many pups are enamored with the contents of the garbage can. While some dogs will quite literally eat anything (we've known dogs to ingest objects ranging from toys to carpets to wood and even lightbulbs), most seek and consume protein-rich foods wherever they can find them. That means that given a choice of foods, most dogs would take the protein-rich option first (then, of course, they'll eat whatever you've got . . .), and

THE VETERINARIAN SAYS

When I was a boy, my brother and I had two Labrador retrievers—Sam was his, and Luke was mine. Once in a while we earned extra money doing chores and went to the store to buy treats for our dogs. At that time, the treat section in the supermarket was about a foot wide, so our choices were easy to make. The same was true of choosing a dog food. For starters, there were only a few to select from, and naturally, we picked the one a smiling Ed McMahon served on *The Tonight Show*. Ed was cool, and his recommendation was good enough for us—besides, the dog he was feeding seemed delighted with the gooey contents of his bowl.

These days, choosing dog foods and treats is much more complicated. Canine nutritional products take up an entire aisle in our grocery store, and there are even more choices available at pet supercenters. While I'm a do-it-yourselfer to the core, when it comes to choosing the best dog food for your pet's needs, I strongly recommend getting the advice of a pro—a veterinarian. It is, I kid you not, literally impossible for the average dog owner to look at the tantalizing ads and competing claims, wade through the ingredients and instructions on a dozen different kinds of dog food, and figure out which is best suited to one dog's needs. Labels are confusing at best, and sometimes just misleading. If you consider the fact that even shoe leather, when laboratory-tested, can technically be assessed as "rich in protein," you'll understand how much room there is for creativity in this area.

This would not be a big issue if all dog foods were created equal, but they are definitely not. When I started out in veterinary practice, one of the first things I learned was that the dogs who came in alert, with bright eyes, high energy, gleaming coats, pleasant doggy smells, and healthy digestive tracts were those that were being fed the correct quantities of recommended premium dog food. Since this one factor has such a substantial tie to your dog's overall health, you shouldn't leave it up to guesswork in the supermarket aisle. Your veterinarian will take into account your dog's breed, age, activity level, current health status, even sexual situation (male, female, sterilized), to recommend the best food and daily amount your dog needs to achieve optimum health. This science-based recommendation of what to put in your pet's bowl will typically change more than five times during your dog's lifetime, starting with puppy food and likely working "up" to senior and prescription diets.

also that they're likely to be extra-enthusiastic and savvy in their efforts to beg for (or steal) meats, cheeses, and similar favorites by any means they have at their disposal.

Born to Run

ODDS are your dog was bred to do a physically demanding job. The American Kennel Club recognizes more than 150 breeds, and well over two-thirds of those were "designed" through selective breeding to perform labors for farmers and hunters. Almost every dog with the word *springer, setter, spaniel, retriever, hound, collie,* or *terrier* in its name falls into one of these categories, as do many, many others. Today, the common denominator among them isn't a role in bringing home their owners' dinner, but a more generic need for exercise to maintain both their physical health and their peace of mind. Dogs who spend their lives sprawled out on (or next to) the couch are highly susceptible to becoming overweight and suffering health implications as a result. The Humane Society of the United States recommends an hour of exercise per day to keep most dogs happy and healthy, regardless of breed. And as is the case with spouses and children, you may have noticed that if your dog isn't happy and healthy, it's difficult for you to achieve that state.

"Stress is the difference between what is and what someone thinks it ought to be," explains Rolan Tripp, DVM, a veterinarian in La Mirada, California, and founder of the Internet resource site animalbehavior.net, "and it's something we often find in dogs who can't figure out why, when they're sure they should be running three to five miles a day, they're cooped up all day long."

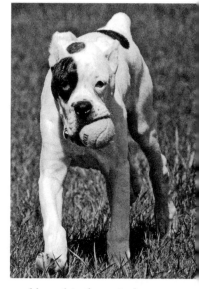

Dr. Tripp's own dogs have long taught him that some breeds get extremely stressed when they don't get their exercise. "My wife and I love Irish setters," he explains, "but they have a reputation for being airheaded, even crazy. Even I was surprised to realize just how much that attitude was caused by cabin fever. As long as our Irish setter gets plenty of exercise, we're dealing with an intelligent, calm, delightful dog."

Just like people, dogs can have all kinds of symptoms that show they're experiencing stresses like what Dr. Tripp calls exercise frustration. Some are pretty obvious about it; they race around the house, jumping around like they've had a triple espresso, or chew inappropriately on the furniture. Others are more subtle. We know dogs who have taken up incessantly grooming themselves, and dogs who act lethargic—depressed really—when they don't get enough exercise. The good news is that most experienced veterinarians and dog-behavior experts agree that there are very few canine behavior problems that cannot be helped—some a little, many a lot—by making sure the dog gets plenty of exercise. The fact is that many stress-related behavior issues can be cleared up completely with a good, long daily walk. As many behaviorists say, "A tired dog is a happy dog!"

To help pinpoint your dog's eating and exercise patterns, take the quiz below. Once you've tallied your answers, you'll find targeted advice on how to help your dog achieve and maintain a healthy weight. And in Chapter 6 we'll explain how you can use these results, and your own, to help unleash fitness for both of you.

Habit Quiz for Pet Participants in the Fitness Unleashed Plan

Part I: Eating Patterns

Circle the answer that best reflects your level of agreement with each statement:

1. My dog has no structured meal routine (same time, place, and amount) from one day to the next.
   a. Not my dog at all. (0 pts)
   b. This is true quite often. (1 pt)
   c. This is my dog most of the time. (2 pts)
   d. That's my dog! (3 pts)

2. The presence of food around my dog triggers him to beg, take a bite, or attempt to wolf it down.
   a. Not my dog at all. (0 pts)
   b. This is true quite often. (1 pt)
   c. This is my dog most of the time. (2 pts)
   d. That's my dog! (3 pts)

3. I have a hard time consistently controlling my dog's portion sizes.
   a. Not at all. (0 pts)
   b. This is true quite often. (1 pt)
   c. This is me most of the time. (2 pts)
   d. That's me. (3 pts)

4. Begging plays a big role in my dog's diet.
   a. Not us at all. (0 pts)
   b. This is true quite often. (1 pt)
   c. This is us most of the time. (2 pts)
   d. That's my dog and I! (3 pts)

5. My dog's snacks are almost all high-calorie treats.
   a. Not my dog at all. (0 pts)
   b. This is true quite often. (1 pt)
   c. This is my dog most of the time. (2 pts)
   d. That's my dog! (3 pts)

6. My dog finds food other than what I put in his bowl by begging, eating the cat's food, scavenging, etc.
   a. Not my dog at all. (0 pts)
   b. This is true quite often. (1 pt)
   c. This is my dog most of the time. (2 pts)
   d. That's my dog! (3 pts)

7. My dog's appetite never seems satiated; he would eat until he exploded if we let him.
   a. Not my dog at all. (0 pts)
   b. This is true quite often. (1 pt)
   c. This is my dog most of the time. (2 pts)
   d. That's my dog! (3 pts)

8. If my dog is slow to eat or refuses to eat a certain food, I'll make it more tasty (toss in some canned food, add gravy, microwave it, etc.) or change diets to a tastier food.
   a. Not at all. (0 pts)
   b. This is true quite often. (1 pt)
   c. This is me most of the time. (2 pts)
   d. That's me (3 pts)

9. My dog gains weight when he's boarded, when someone house-sits, or when we have company because he's so good at getting people to give him treats.
   a. Not my dog at all. (0 pts)
   b. This is true quite often. (1 pt)
   c. This is my dog most of the time. (2 pts)
   d. That's my dog! (3 pts)

10. I make sure my dog has food in his bowl at all times.
   a. Not at all. (0 pts)
   b. This is true quite often. (1 pt)
   c. This is me most of the time. (2 pts)
   d. That's me. (3 pts)

11. I often share my own snacks and treats with my dog. He loves ice cream (or buttered popcorn or oatmeal cookies) as much as I do.
   a. Not at all. (0 pts)
   b. This is true quite often. (1 pt)
   c. This is me most of the time. (2 pts)
   d. That's me. (3 pts)

12. My dog knows just how to push my buttons to get an extra treat. If you saw the way he works those puppy-dog eyes, you'd feed him extra, too.

a. Not my dog at all. (0 pts)

b. This is true quite often. (1 pt)

c. This is my dog most of the time. (2 pts)

d. That's my dog! (3 pts)

Here's How to Score Your Dog's Eating Habits:

Add points from questions 5, 8, and 11 to get a
SPOILED SNACKER score: _____

Add points from questions 2, 6, and 7 to get a
GARBAGE GUT score: _____

Add points from questions 4, 9, and 12 to get a
SHAMELESS BEGGAR score: _____

Add points from questions 1, 3, and 10 to get a
FREE FEEDER score: _____

The highest total score reveals your dog's dominant eating-personality type. If there's a tie among the highest scores, then pick the eating pattern that you feel fits your dog best. Each pattern description below includes steps you can take to make sure your pup is getting enough, but not too much, to eat.

Eating Patterns

SPOILED SNACKER

What a lucky dog this is: loved and pampered and given all the perks of full family-member status. Congratulations on having such a solid, affectionate relationship with your dog. Now we must tell you, as many a doting parent has had to learn, that it's easy to mingle food and love, offering treats as signs of your affection—but that practice is generally not good for your dog's health. If your dog is overweight, try taking these simple steps to help him get lean.

1. Cut treats in half. Dogs who regularly receive treats in addition to their meals are 50 percent more likely to be overweight than those who don't. To save both you and your dog from suffering during treat cutbacks, we suggest you start off by cutting your treat offerings in half. Simply take whatever goody your dog is accustomed to getting and split it in two—half for today, half for tomorrow. That way, your dog will still get the same attention and sense of reward from you, but for half the calories.

2. Show your affection in action. You may think your dog would be miserable if you stopped sharing treats with him, but we're willing to bet he would be happy to accept a substitute. Think of a favorite activity or game your dog enjoys playing with you—or make one up. We know one dog owner who plays a made-up game that combines hide-and-seek and tag for a few minutes with his poodle every night after work. The dog gets so excited about this daily game that he starts "hiding," lying in wait behind the coffee table, as soon as the car pulls into the driveway. A short, scheduled playtime is a great substitute for a shared treat anytime.

3. Substitute talk for treats. While we all know dogs love to do the furry tap dance at the sight, smell, or taste of treats, fewer of us understand and appreciate how tantalizing talk can be to a dog. They simply lap it up when we baby-talk to them, get animated, and act silly. For years Dr. Becker has recommended clients give their pets lots and lots of "emotional Milk-Bones." Many have been shocked at how readily their dogs accept this kind of audible "treat" instead of an edible one.

NOT-FOR-DOGS FOODS

Many pet owners enjoy offering their dogs tidbits of "people food," and in some places in this book we recommend it. It's important to be aware, though, that some foods for humans can be potentially harmful to dogs. The ASPCA Animal Poison Control Center advises against giving pets the following foods:

Chocolate—Chocolate can cause intestinal irritation, hyperactivity, panting, abnormal heart rhythm, tremors, and seizures.

Xylitol—Candy, gum, and other products containing large amounts of the sweetener xylitol can cause a rapid drop in blood sugar, resulting in depression, loss of coordination, and seizures.

Coffee—Coffee can produce the same effects as chocolate, depending on the dose.

Fatty foods—Foods high in fat can cause stomach upset.

Moldy or spoiled foods—If you're tossing food from the fridge and Fido is hanging around looking for a bite, keep in mind that some rotting foods can make dogs sick, too.

Onions—Onions, garlic, and chives can produce intestinal upset and can cause damage to red blood cells.

Salt (including foods high in salt)—Salt and foods containing large quantities of salt can produce sodium-ion poisoning in dogs.

Macadamia nuts—Macadamias can produce weakness (particularly in the hind legs), and severe illness in dogs.

Raisins and grapes—These surprising culprits have been associated with acute kidney failure in some dogs.

Yeast dough—Yeast-based dough can not only expand in the GI tract as it rises, causing an intestinal obstruction, but the yeast can form alcohol when it rises, which can cause alcohol poisoning.

Tomato—While the red, ripe fruit is not considered to be toxic, the leaves, stem, and green unripe fruit can cause stomach upset, drowsiness, weakness, and slow heart rate.

Potato—As they are in the same family as the tomato, the green plant parts of the potato can produce similar effects.

4. Choose treats you can feel good about. Your dog may be accustomed to dog treats that look like miniature steaks, pieces of cheese, and Fig Newtons, but if you really want to share your food with him, he'd be far better off eating bits of fruits and vegetables instead. This might sound silly, but we've never met a dog yet who doesn't enjoy at least one fruit or veggie treat. A few favorites we've seen are whole baby carrots, frozen green beans or peas, blueberries, and apple slices. You may be surprised to find that your dog also enjoys broccoli, bananas, or even lettuce. Try a few of these low-calorie, nutrient-rich options and let your dog choose for himself. Unlike small children, most dogs aren't especially susceptible to choking. If your dog (or more likely, your puppy) chokes on a particular food, though, either cut it into smaller pieces or choose a different treat altogether.

GARBAGE GUT

This dog is so hungry! Everything is fair game, and nothing is ever enough. This dog will tear open a trash bag and eat not just the food inside, but also anything with a little food on it. He'll chew through plastic, paper, cardboard, and in extreme circumstances drywall to get to a meal. You've probably seen this dog all but hyperventilate as he watches you prepare his meal—and maybe also yours. This dog's body has no discernible "fullness detector" and he will literally eat himself sick whenever the circumstances allow. The gluttony is really not his fault—just a genetic predisposition to making sure he never starves to death and always has enough calories to feed his busy lifestyle. Naturally, the odds are this big eater is a dog who requires plenty of exercise, too.

1. Outwit and outmaneuver. If your dog is really a Dumpster-diver and a food-on-counter-stealer, you're going to have to beat him at his own game to reduce his calorie intake. The first step is just accepting that this is a problem that affects your dog's health and that it needs to be dealt with. Perhaps if Rover has been augmenting his diet by helping himself to the all-you-can-eat garbage buffet for a long time, you've come to accept this as the way things are. Try one of the following to break your dog's bad habit:

- Sprinkle on baking powder. Most dogs have a favorite time of day (or night) for trash-can raids. Before bed or before your dog's trash time, generously sprinkle the top of the trash in the bin with baking powder. While some dogs enjoy hot pepper sauce and other spices people use as repellants to keep them out of the trash, very few will keep eating beyond the icky taste of the alum in baking powder. Even though it's unappetizing and should help curb the problem, it won't hurt your dog if he eats some.

- Buy a lid lock. Toddler-proof garbage-can lid locks available in any discount store are even more effective in keeping dogs out of the trash than they are in keeping kids out. This inexpensive solution will bring your dog's garbage-can raid to a quick halt.

- Prepare food in a dog-safe area. If you have a big dog, you may also have experienced the theft of food off the kitchen counter and table. You can find a useful tool in preventing counter theft in the toddler aisle. Oven guards are clear plastic shields that will block your dog from reaching food on countertops. They are inexpensive and easy to remove once you break your dog of his bad habit.

2. Spread meals across the day. One of the best ways to make sure your dog isn't truly suffering from hunger is to split up his meals so he gets to eat more than once a day. A two- or up to

four-times-a-day eating plan is healthier and more satisfying for your dog. If, in fact, your dog has been consuming lots of calories on the sly, you may even be able to up his daily dose of kibble once you've gotten his snacking habit under control. Ask the veterinarian how much food your dog should have daily, divide it into equal portions, and stick with the plan.

SHAMELESS BEGGAR

Those wide eyes. Those perked ears. That wagging tail. Your dog may deserve an Academy Award for his gifts in working any audience for a treat. We're always amazed at how an accomplished beggar dog can change his routine to suit his potential treat giver. To his primary caretaker, he looks like he really just needs one more bite. To the kids in the house, he looks like he'll turn somersaults for just one teeny-tiny nibble of whatever they're having. To well-meaning neighbors and guests, he fixes his best "Can't you see they're not feeding me here?" look in hopes of a big score. This dog has talent, and his unique abilities are getting him into big trouble. Here's how to shut down the effectiveness of this treat-scoring machine.

1. Enact a permanent ban on treats from the table. Many of the goodies that dogs successfully beg for come straight from the family table. Eliminating this one area of begging will likely cut down substantially on your dog's treat quota. If you're going to have a hard time sticking with a decision not to share table food, we suggest putting your dog in another room, in his crate, or out in the backyard during mealtimes. If you really want to share a healthy scrap of your own food with your

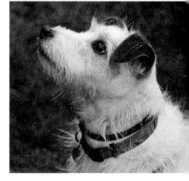

dog, you still can—just put it in his bowl instead of offering it under the table.

2. Get your family, friends, and neighbors on the plan. An effective Shameless Beggar is like a con artist in search of a dupe. Anyone who will give in is an ideal target; they'll eat three squares a day at your house and squeeze in a few more off the pet-loving neighbor's patio. When you decide to turn off your dog's begging, be sure your entire family is on board, as well as any friends, neighbors, pet sitters, or other caregivers who interact with him.

3. Try a beg-and-switch policy. What would happen if every time your dog begged for a sausage or a bone he was rewarded with a baby carrot or a snap pea? One of two things: your dog will either cut down on his begging or develop a taste for a fresh vegetable. Either one of those would be good, wouldn't it?

4. Share time instead. When your dog starts begging, take a minute to play fetch or chase or to tickle his tummy or rub his ears. One of the things that surprised many of the participants in the PPET study was that there was no increase in begging behaviors as their dogs started receiving less food and more walks. It seemed the extra exercise and attention was an acceptable substitute.

FREE FEEDER

When we talk about this doggie dining personality, owners of certain breeds (Labs and beagles come to mind) inevitably laugh and point out that if they free-fed their dogs, those dogs would literally eat themselves to death. We know of one 90-pound dog who, left alone in the garage with a full bag of dog food for the day, polished off the entire 40 pounds. Yuck! In fact, this category is for dogs who do *not* blatantly make pigs of themselves, but who are routinely given more food and more time to eat it than they need. These are dogs like Clancy, a corgi belonging to Matilda Murphy in Bethlehem, Pennsylvania. When given 2 cups of food in the morning, Clancy spends about five minutes eating half, then walks away. Half an hour later, he often goes back for more, and then hits the bowl again one more time to finish off the food. It may sound like this is a dog who just enjoys his kibble, but in fact, it's a dog who is receiving too much.

1. Measure or weigh, every day. The significant problem with the Free Feeder's diet is that it's not consistent—or that it's consistently too much. We recommend the next time you're at the grocery store you invest in a 1-cup measure to be used from today on to measure your dog's food. Next, put in a call to or visit your dog's veterinarian to ask how much of what food is the ideal amount for each day. Divide that quantity into two or three portions, and feed your dog only the measured amount.

   While there is no substitute for a veterinarian's recommendation about what food and how much your dog needs, we've seen enough clients who are far, far off the mark to want to offer a basic guideline so you know if you're in the right ballpark. Dr. Steve Garner, a veterinarian in League City, Texas, and owner of Safari Animal Care Center, explains the science and math of dog-food portions better than anyone we know:

   "As a rule of thumb, dogs come in three sizes: small, medium, and large, each with different caloric needs. In general, a small dog needs forty calories per pound of body weight per day, a medium-sized dog needs thirty calories per pound, and a large dog needs only twenty calories per pound. So if you multiply the dog's weight by the correct number of calories per pound, you'll get a rough idea of what that dog needs to con-

DOGGY DIET FOOD

If your dog is overweight and you're having difficulty helping him take off the extra pounds (either because he seems not to be getting enough to eat when you cut back on the regular food, or perhaps because you've cut back his allotment and he's still gaining), talk with your veterinarian about the possibility of feeding him a prescription-diet food. All the canine participants in the PPET study ate Hill's Prescription Diet Canine r/d food at the same time they undertook the walking program, and their weight-loss results were excellent. In fact, the dogs substantially outperformed the human participants in the measure of percentage of body weight lost.

Prescription-diet dog foods are not just "light" versions of regular foods, but different formulations designed to help meet your dog's nutritional needs—and help him feel full—on fewer calories. Veterinarian-recommended brands have been described as "tastes great, more filling" reduced-calorie alternatives.

sume to maintain a healthy weight (for example, a thirty-pound dog times thirty calories per pound per day equals nine hundred calories a day).

"Most dry dog foods contain an average of 350 calories per measuring cup—so that same thirty-pound dog would require slightly less than three measuring cups of food a day. Because canned food is mostly water, most brands contain about half as many calories per cup as dry food, so the allotment for the thirty-pound dog would be more."

Dr. Garner's formula will help you determine if you're substantially overfeeding or underfeeding your dog, but he cautions that the numbers above are just a guideline—some dog foods have more or fewer calories per cup—and that the only way to be sure your dog is getting the right amount of food is to monitor his body weight or ask your veterinarian for guidance.

2. Same time, same place. To further ensure you're in control of how much your dog eats and when, feed him at the same time and in the same place whenever you can. A set schedule gives your dog a clear sense of when the next meal is coming. It'll alleviate any need he may feel to "save something for later."

3. Pick up the bowl. Give your dog ten to fifteen minutes with his food at each meal, then pick up the bowl with any food left in it. We don't recommend that you pick up the bowl the minute your dog is finished, because it may make him feel like he's got to wolf down his meals or lose them; but after ten minutes, your dog has eaten all he needs of any given meal. Any kibble left over is just going to contribute extra, unneeded calories.

Part II: Exercise Patterns

Circle the answer that best reflects your level of agreement with each statement:

1. If my dog doesn't get enough exercise, he does things like dig holes in the yard, bark too much, chew up household items, or nervously pace by the door.
   a. Not my dog at all. (0 pts)
   b. This is true quite often. (1 pt)
   c. This is my dog most of the time. (2 pts)
   d. That's my dog! (3 pts)

2. I seldom walk my dog because of his osteoarthritis, hip dysplasia, lethargy, low stamina, or other medical condition.
   a. Not at all. (0 pts)
   b. This is true quite often. (1 pt)
   c. This is me most of the time. (2 pts)
   d. That's me. (3 pts)

3. My dog is equally happy parked on the couch or speed-walking through the park, as long as he's with me.
   a. Not my dog at all. (0 pts)
   b. This is true quite often. (1 pt)
   c. This is my dog most of the time. (2 pts)
   d. That's my dog! (3 pts)

4. My dog's behavior definitely takes a turn for the worse if he doesn't get a walk for a day or more.
   a. Not my dog at all. (0 pts)
   b. This is true quite often. (1 pt)
   c. This is my dog most of the time. (2 pts)
   d. That's my dog! (3 pts)

5. My dog is too small, too chubby, or too old to walk for twenty minutes or more a day.
   a. Not my dog at all. (0 pts)
   b. This is true quite often. (1 pt)
   c. This is my dog most of the time. (2 pts)
   d. That's my dog! (3 pts)

6. My dog would rather sleep than walk or chase a tennis ball.
   a. Not my dog at all. (0 pts)
   b. This is true quite often. (1 pt)
   c. This is my dog most of the time. (2 pts)
   d. That's my dog! (3 pts)

7. My dog likes to walk and play, but he's just as happy to hang out around the house.
   a. Not my dog at all. (0 pts)
   b. This is true quite often. (1 pt)
   c. This is my dog most of the time. (2 pts)
   d. That's my dog! (3 pts)

8. It's been at least a week since the last time I walked my dog for twenty minutes or more.
   a. Not at all. (0 pts)
   b. This is true quite often. (1 pt)
   c. This is me most of the time. (2 pts)
   d. That's me. (3 pts)

9. My dog could walk or run or chase a tennis ball forever. I rarely see any signs of limits to his energy.
   a. Not my dog at all. (0 pts)
   b. This is true quite often. (1 pt)
   c. This is my dog most of the time. (2 pts)
   d. That's my dog! (3 pts)

10. I don't exercise my dog much because I'm afraid I might push him too hard or that the effort could hurt him.
    a. Not at all. (0 pts)
    b. This is true quite often. (1 pt)
    c. This is me most of the time. (2 pts)
    d. That's me. (3 pts)

11. My dog might sleep the day (and the night) away if he didn't have to get up to eat and go outside to relieve himself.
    a. Not my dog at all. (0 pts)
    b. This is true quite often. (1 pt)
    c. This is my dog most of the time. (2 pts)
    d. That's my dog! (3 pts)

12. When I'm on an exercise kick, so is my dog; but if I'm on a stay-inside-and-take-it-easy kick, my dog loves to live that lifestyle, too.

   a. Not my dog at all. (0 pts)

   b. This is true quite often. (1 pt)

   c. This is my dog most of the time. (2 pts)

   d. That's my dog! (3 pts)

Here's How to Score Your Dog's Exercise Habits:

Add points from question 1, 4, and 9 to get an
ENERGIZER PUP score: _____

Add points from questions 6, 8, and 11 to get a
PASSIVE POOCH score: _____

Add points from questions 3, 7, and 12 to get a
GOOD BUDDY score: _____

Add points from questions 2, 5, and 10 to get a
FRAGILE FIDO score: _____

The highest total score reveals your pet's dominant exercise-personality type. If there's a tie among the highest scores, then pick the pattern that you think best fits. See pattern descriptions below.

Exercise Patterns

ENERGIZER PUP

If this dog could talk, he might tell you, with remarkably little malice intended, "If I don't get enough exercise, I'll make your life miserable." He might be a bigger dog, maybe a breed with *retriever* or *setter* or *collie* in his name. He may or may not be an actual "puppy," but he certainly acts like one at even the hint of a walk or a game of fetch. Whether he's a purebred or a mixed-breed dog, his ancestors were bred to be high-energy hard workers. There's a good chance a short daily walk doesn't make a dent in this dog's needs for exercise, and you may even find he has more energy when you get home than he did when you started out. It takes a little extra creativity to meet the exercise needs of a dog like this, but in Chapter 6 we'll show you exactly how to wear out your Energizer Pup without running yourself ragged. If you're embarking on the Fitness Unleashed program to help lose weight off your own frame, too, you've got an incredible, motivating workout partner in this dog. Once he knows your routine, he's never going to let you forget, postpone, or cut corners again.

PASSIVE POOCH

At the opposite end of the spectrum is the dog who just loves to lie around. Maggie Morgan, who lives in West Michigan, lovingly described her golden retriever, Holly, as a docile girl and a "living rug" before they undertook an exercise regimen together. "Holly moves slowly, she's gentle, and she's a great big armful to hug," says Maggie smiling. It's all too easy to let a dog like this lie—after all, sweet, docile dogs are the ideal pet for many of us, and we don't want to stir up a good thing. Unfortunately, with that lifestyle comes extra weight. "There's a poster on the wall at our veterinary office that illustrates the various states of health for dogs, from severely undernourished to extremely overweight," Morgan explains. "Maggie has reached the 'no waistline' stage of that chart, and if she keeps gaining at her current rate, she'll resemble the last 'bulging at the waist' photo before long. Her veterinarian says she has to lose at least eight pounds."

Your goal is to motivate your Passive Pooch to get moving and to stick to a routine. This dog may never want to tag along on a ten-mile hike with you, but we're willing to bet you can use our tips in

Chapter 7, "Making It Fun for Fido" to get him off the couch and excited to head out with you.

GOOD BUDDY

This dog will take exercise or leave it, as long as you're happy. He's game for a walk, and equally into a ball game and a bowl of popcorn on the couch. If you choose a sedentary lifestyle for the two of you to share, well, this dog's not going to complain about it. Instead, he's going to become overweight, and over time, he's likely to develop obesity-related health problems that could make him uncomfortable and even shorten his life. Rather than let that happen, we think you should enlist this exemplary, easygoing Man's Best Friend as your exercise partner and let both your health and his health benefit as a result. In Chapter 6, we'll tell you exactly how to get this dog on board with a new fitness program. We guarantee your Good Buddy can quickly learn to be as punctual and reliable as an alarm clock in getting both of you out the door to exercise.

FRAGILE FIDO

Too old, too young, too small, too infirm. This dog may have physical limitations like arthritis, hip dysplasia, or sensitivity to heat or cold that discourage you from taking him for walks. It may even be that your dog isn't getting much exercise due to soreness or sluggishness because of excess weight. Even though there are many legitimate reasons to carefully regulate or pace some dogs' exercise, the fact is that even those who are elderly and infirm

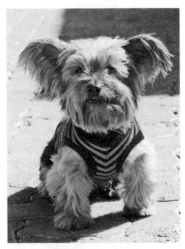

can greatly benefit from the opportunity to walk. In Chapter 6, we'll show you just how to start your dog on a slow-and-steady program of life-extending, health-enhancing exercise.

We know these pattern assessments can't fully capture the unique charms and personalities of your one-of-a-kind dog, but they do help you take a hard look at the reasons he may be gaining weight and losing fitness. In the next chapter, we'll show you how to take the first steps in reclaiming your dog's health and fitness—and how to start doing the same for yourself.

CHAPTER 5

Ready, Set:
Starting Out on the
Right Foot (or Paw)

Walking is so wonderful—it's as safe and effective an exercise program as any you'll ever find, and it works equally well for both you and your dog. And despite the health and weight-loss benefits it offers, walking requires less preparation, less equipment, and less investment in general than any sport we can think of. There are a few factors, though, that can make a significant difference in how well a walking program works. To help you both set off on the "right" foot, we've put together the following seven steps to take the week before you begin in earnest. You can do one a day, if you like, for a steady ramp-up to the program.

1. Learn to Play the Numbers Game

ONE of the keys to effectively using a walking program for weight loss (yours or your dog's) is getting an accurate assessment of how long and how far you walk each day—not just when you're working out, but from the time you get out of bed in the morning until the time you get back in at night. So, before you do anything else, get a pedometer and review the instructions about how to use it. Pedometers come in tons of varieties, from the very complex with features like radios, clocks, and personal alarms to simple step counters. Any pedometer that accurately counts your steps is fine. At the Wellness Institute, we've found the ones from the Accusplit company (you can view their products at accusplit.com) to be among the most consistently accurate.

Like any piece of equipment, the pedometer needs to be used properly if it's going to work. First, know where to wear it. The pedometer should be worn on your waistband or belt roughly in line with your foot on either side of your body. Be sure that the pedometer is fastened snugly on the belt or waistband. Many of them come with a leash that clips on a belt loop for extra security. For women who wear clothes without a belt or waistband, try wearing it fastened onto your undergarments. Second, make sure it counts what it's supposed to. After setting the pedometer to zero and closing the cover, take 100 steps and count them out in your head. Stop and check the pedometer reading. If it registers between 95 and 105 steps, you're ready to go. (When you're consistently walking for an extended period, this margin of error that appears to be 5 percent will go down. Many counters tend to count a couple steps high or low when you first start walking as they adjust to your gait. As you continue moving, their accuracy will improve.) If your step count for 100 steps is off by more than 5 paces, try readjusting the pedometer on your belt or waistband an inch or two to the right or left and check again. It's a good idea to repeat the walking-test calibration on a weekly to monthly basis.

Once you've figured out how to work your new counter, clip it on and wear it all day for at least three days. Keep it on for everything

A "PET"OMETER, TOO?

No, your dog doesn't need his own *"pet*-ometer," but yes, they make one. This gizmo, from Spot Pets, Inc., clips onto your dog's collar and measures actual distance traveled (not steps taken) for your dog. It accounts for your dog's size and stride to get as accurate a measurement as possible. (A recent study published in the *Journal of the American Veterinary Medical Association* showed that while pet-ometers are not 100 percent accurate, they do work well enough to measure a dog's physical activity with reasonable accuracy.) The pedometer you wear will keep track of the distance you and your dog travel together, but if you've ever wondered just how much ground your pooch covers running loops around you or racing after a tennis ball again and again in the park (or maybe you've wondered just how little your dog walks when it seems like he's sacked out in the living room all of the time), then this is the gadget for you.

but bathing and swimming. Choose days that are representative of your activity level (for example, two weekdays and one weekend day during which you follow your normal routine). Many pedometers measure distance covered and calories burned, but the number you're looking for is simply steps taken. Every night when you unclip the pedometer, write down your total steps for the day and reset the pedometer to zero for the next day. After the third day, add all three step counts and divide by three; the average of these numbers is your baseline step count for Fitness Unleashed. You may find you're walking just 2,000 or 3,000 steps a day, or if your days are more active, you may cover 6,000 or more. One of the great advantages of the Fitness Unleashed program is that it starts at your current exertion level. No matter how many steps you're walking right now, we'll show you in the next chapter how to maximize the program.

2. Choose Your Shoes

THE single most important piece of equipment you need for this exercise program (besides your dog!) is a good pair of walking shoes. From the ankles up, you can wear whatever makes you happy while sticking to your new routine (most people prefer comfortable, breathable, freely moving clothes). From the ankles down, please follow our advice for choosing shoes that will help support your frame and prevent injuries:

● Get the right type. There are so many kinds of athletic shoes on the market, it's easy to think that any of them will work for an activity as basic as walking. For the occasional walker, that's probably true, but as you undertake a regular walking program, you'll need to be more selective. Shoes designed for running, walking, or cross-training are your best bet. We recommend you stay away from shoes designed for other sports—especially shoes designed for court sports like basketball and tennis. Court shoes are designed to allow for side-to-side foot movement, and so they aren't suitable for distance walking.

According to the American Orthopaedic Foot and Ankle Society, a good walking shoe is one with a soft upper, plenty of cushioning for good shock absorption, and a rocker sole design that encourages the natural roll of your foot during the walking motion.

● When trying on shoes, ask for a half size bigger than you wear in street shoes. There should be about a quarter-inch of "wiggle room" between the end of your toe and the wall of the shoe. While you do want room in the toes, the heel should fit snugly with very little room for back-and-forth movement. If your heel is not secure in the shoe, your feet can get chafed or blistered—the last thing any walker wants.

● Be sure you try both shoes! Your feet may not be the exact same size. This is especially important if this is your first pair of exercise shoes in a while.

● Choose the ones that fit. As we age, our feet can change size and shape quite a bit (most often getting wider)—so a pair of shoes that would have fit perfectly five years ago may not fit at all today. Also, any pair of shoes that's going to be comfortable enough for you to wear to walk in five days a week will feel good on your feet while you're still in the shoe store. If they feel like they need to be "broken in" or stretched out, choose another pair.

● Unlike a pair of dress shoes for a night on the town, your walking shoes have no margin for discomfort. If you're buying a new pair, before you make a selection, take them for a trial walk. If the salesperson won't let you take them around the block (many will—as will almost any store that specializes in running shoes), make a few laps around the shop to make sure there are no points of pressure or chafing for your feet.

● Talk with the salesperson about arch support. For a first pair of walking shoes, it's probably worth your trouble to go to a shoe store that specializes in running shoes so you'll get the help of a salesclerk who knows how to help you get the right fit and support.

● A word about socks. (Actually, two words . . .) Thorlo, Coolmax. Socks made of one of these patented blended fab-

THE ULTIMATE ACCESSORY

If you're a parent to an infant or a small child, that "accessory" can be a cute kid in a stroller on your dog walks. Don't let the dual responsibilities of managing stroller and leash deter you, as both can definitely be handled. We know one mom who loops the end of the leash around the handle of a jogging stroller and lets her Lab help pull both stroller and baby up the steep hills on her route. For ease of pushing the baby, you might also considering making the small investment in a hands-free leash (available at pet-supply stores).

rics are widely recommended by both fitness and foot experts because they're far more efficient at keeping your feet dry and comfortable while you're walking than socks made of just cotton.

3. Outfit Your Dog

THE right leash and collar are as important to your dog's health and safety as a good pair of shoes is for you. Unless you have a dog trained to come on command with 100 percent reliability and you live in an area with no neighbors and no traffic, we strongly recommend keeping your dog on a leash at all times as you begin your walking routine together. Even a well-trained dog can get excited at the sight of a squirrel or another dog or somebody's sandwich wrapper, and you don't want to have to worry about your dog wandering away or getting into trouble. Studies show owners report pulling on

THE VETERINARIAN SAYS: THE NAILS HAVE IT

You and your dog are cruising along down the sidewalk, side by side, breathing deeply and enjoying the morning sun or an afternoon breeze. In a quiet moment, the only sound is the "click, click, click" of your dog's nails as they tap against the pavement.

Wait, wait, wait! Before you take another step (or at least another walk), trim those toenails! If you can hear your dog's nails as he moves, they're too long. In fact, with every step, they're pushing back into his toes, causing him to roll or rotate his foot to compensate. Imagine yourself taking a walk while trying to hold a dime between your toes and you'll get a sense of how walking with overlong toenails throws off your dog's gait.

Nail trimming can be easily and safely done at home with a nail clipper designed for dogs (be sure to get one for the right-sized dog—most are labeled for small, medium, or large dogs). However, if either you or your workout buddy is not comfortable with this arrangement, have the veterinarian's office or a groomer handle the trimming. This quick, inexpensive step will help ensure your dog's comfort—and safety—while walking.

the leash and lunging as the number-one problems in walking their dogs. Follow these guidelines to get your pet outfitted for your adventure together:

THE COLLAR

In outfitting your dog for the new walking routine, do as Stephen Covey describes in *The 7 Habits of Highly Effective People,* and "begin with the end in mind." If you begin with the right anchor point(s) on the dog, you'll end up with a pet that's easy to walk.

Select a snap or buckle, nylon or leather collar that can be adjusted to properly fit your dog's neck. It should be small enough that it can't possibly slide over your dog's head, and otherwise be as loose as possible. A new choice is the Premier martingale-type collar, which prevents a dog from escaping by backing out of the collar or wriggling it off.

We also recommend a product called the Gentle Leader Easy Walk Harness as a collar alternative to have control and safety while walking your dog. Unlike collars, the Easy Walk Harness prevents pulling and lunging without causing coughing, gagging, or choking, because the chest strap rests low across the breastbone instead of on the delicate trachea at the front of the throat. The harness's chest attachment stops your dog from pulling by steering to the side, provides extra leverage for relaxed control, and works wonders in redirecting the dog's attention to you.

If you feel you need additional control for excessive pulling or to stem behaviors like lunging, jumping, and bark-

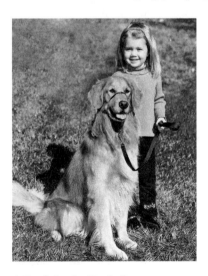

A Gentle Leader Headcollar

PRONG COLLARS AND CHOKE CHAINS

Because these two varieties of collars are so often misused, we don't recommend either one without the supervision of a dog trainer. However, if you're certain you want to use one or the other, choose the prong collar over a choke collar. Collars that simply tighten around a dog's neck are not particularly effective in getting the dog to follow commands or walk properly, and they pose a health risk to your dog, as they can all too easily damage his neck or affect his breathing.

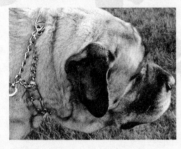

A prong collar

With spikes around the inside that apply pressure to a dog's neck when he pulls against the leash, the medieval-looking prong collar may appear awfully unfriendly, but it's actually less likely to hurt a dog than a regular choke collar, explains Sophia Yin, DVM, applied animal behaviorist and coinventor of the Treat & Train Positive Reinforcement Dog Training System. This is because the pressure from a tug on the prong collar is distributed over a larger area on the dog—rather than focused on the dog's windpipe.

If you're going to use either of these collars, consider Dr. Yin's advice for doing so correctly and effectively:

Remember that all training should be more about praise than punishment. When your dog is doing the right thing, praise him. When he's walking nicely on the leash, give him a small treat as you keep going. This teaches him to *keep* behaving well. When your dog starts doing something you don't want him to do, give a sharp, strong, quick correction with the collar. You want your dog to be very clear about which behavior is unacceptable.

The primary problem with prong collars, Dr. Yin explains, is that when many owners use them, they're thinking only about punishment. Keep in mind that the ratio of praise to punishment in any kind of dog training should be 20 to 1 or higher.

ing, we recommend using a head halter like the Gentle Leader Headcollar. The Headcollar works like a halter on a horse, with a loop that rests over the dog's nose, to guide and control any size dog without pressure on the throat. If your dog does surge forward—that darned squirrel or squirrely little dog darts by again—the Headcollar will give you control without choking. Because this product mimics the pressure a mother dog would apply to the top of a pup's snout, many pet owners who use it find that it also has a calming, reassuring effect on shy, nervous dogs. For more information on either Gentle Leader product, visit www.premier.com.

○ We know you love this dog, so make absolutely sure that if the two of you ever get separated on a walk, you'll be able to get him back quickly and safely. The best way to ensure that happy reunion is by making sure your dog is easily identifiable as a beloved member of *your* family. Be sure he has an identification tag attached to his collar with his name and your phone numbers. Unfortunately, ID tags often become detached, so also use a Sharpie to write a contact number directly on your dog's nylon or leather collar. Last but not least, we strongly recommend you go to your local veterinarian to get the latest ISO identification microchip for dogs. The implantable microchip—the size of a grain of rice—is inserted between your dog's shoulder blades, and it is no more painful than a routine vaccination. Once it's been implanted, if your dog is picked up by animal control and taken to a veterinarian or a local animal shelter, the chip can be instrumental in getting him back home to you. Pardon the pun, but as one out of three dogs is lost sometime in its life, there's a good chance that someday your pet's "chip will come in" and you'll have a happy, slobbery reunion.

WHAT TO DO WHEN YOUR DOG THINKS HIS COLLAR IS A PAIN IN THE NECK

There are generally two kinds of dogs who don't get along with collars and leashes: puppies and adult dogs who have never worn them before, and dogs who are breaking in new collars. Either way, here's how to help him get used to his new accessory.

● First and foremost, make sure there's no good reason for the complaint. Take off the collar and run your hand carefully along the inside of it (the part that comes in contact with your dog's neck). Is it completely smooth? If the fabric is uneven or scratchy, consider replacing the collar completely. Next, put on the collar and make sure it's not too tight. If the fit isn't right, take it off and adjust it in your hands (not while it's around your dog's neck).

● As you put on the collar, give your dog a treat. Once it's on and set, give him another. Then, ignore him. Wearing a collar for the first time is a lot like wearing a wedding ring; it feels funny at first, *and* it represents a long-term relationship at the other end of a leash. Your dog needs a chance to get used to the feeling.

● When your dog stops rolling and rubbing and scratching at the collar, attach the leash and let the dog drag the leash inside the house. If he follows you from room to room, give him treats for sticking nearby with the leash on.

● Next, take the dog into your yard, pick up the leash, and just follow the dog around praising him wherever he goes. You want your dog to be thinking something along the lines of, "Where has this leash been all my life?"

● Before long (somewhere between one hour and one day for most dogs) the leash is going to be old news, and most dogs will fall right into step once they get used to it. If your dog continues to resist being walked on a lead, turn to Chapter 7, "Making It Fun for Fido," for tips on making your walking partnership enjoyable for both of you.

THE LEASH

Once you've settled on the right collar, choosing the right leash is a piece of cake. If your dog is making the adjustment to being tethered to you (see page 119), use a four-foot leash to make this transition. The short length gives your dog less to get tangled with during the drag-the-leash-from-room-to-room period, and less for him to trip on when you do pick up the other end.

Once your dog gets over objecting to his leash and collar, though, we recommend a retractable lead for almost any walk. If you live in a city, be aware that there may be an ordinance that dictates maximum leash length, and you'll need to abide by this, particularly when in the vicinity of other people. If this is the case for you, you might choose a retractable with a maximum length of ten feet. If you have more room to roam and no civic limitations, though, choose a lead with a longer full-extension length—sixteen feet or more. You can always choose to keep it short as needed, but the wiggle room that comes with the extendable leash will let your dog do more exploring while you keep walking—a win-win situation. The fact that the leash reels itself up as the dog comes closer to you will save you many stops along the way to untangle his feet from a loose lead. One caution, though: We recommend using a wrist strap (available in pet supply stores) to help secure the retractable lead, as it is easier to drop than a standard leash.

4. Take a Wide-Eyed Look at Your World

TURN your attention to your friends and family, your coworkers, and your pantry. Every house and every circle of friends comes equipped with a few pitfalls to your best intentions to lose weight and get fit. Ask the people you trust for their support in your new endeavor—specific requests like "Please don't bring any more

LEASH FOR TWO

If you're walking two dogs and finding yourself all tied up between two leashes, we've got a great product for you! The Tangle-Me-Knot leash is designed with a split end to connect to two collars and a swivel base so the dogs can cross behind and in front of one another without completely throwing you off. You can check it out in pet stores or at www.tobzpet.com.

doughnuts to my desk"; "Could you watch the kids for half an hour on Thursday night while I walk?"; or "When the dog wants a treat, reach for the baby carrots" will help bring them on board with your new program. You've got an ideal, built-in workout partner in your dog, but the more social support you have, the better.

Next, take the time to clear high-calorie, low-nutrition foods like chips, cookies, ice cream, and soda out of your house. *No* foods are forbidden in Fitness Unleashed, but not having these items at home will make them treats, not staples. Stock up on items from our list of flavorful, more healthful alternatives.

5. Get the Official A-Okay

BECAUSE walking is such gentle exercise, it may not be necessary to get clearance from your doctor (or your dog's veterinarian) to start this program. However, if you have any history of health ailments that have limited your level of activity, this is the time to speak

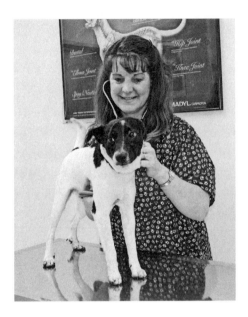

with your doctor about your intention to begin regular dog walks of gradually increasing distance and intensity.

If your dog has a history of health problems, is out of shape, or is under six months or over seven years old, check in with the veterinarian, too, to make sure you're starting off at the right pace. Any dog with a history of cardiac, pulmonary, or joint problems should definitely have a visit with the vet before starting any exercise program.

6. Know How to Walk Safely

ONE of us recently saw a greeting card with a picture of a very elderly lady with a cane on the front and a caption that read, "To maintain my girlish figure and mental agility, I walk five miles a day." Inside the card, in large, crooked letters was the exclamation, "Now where the heck am I??"

We've been saying since page 1 that walking is safe, and it is, but taking certain basic precautions—including knowing your route well enough to ensure you never get lost—can make it even more risk free for you and your dog.

The most basic rules of safe walking are the ones you've likely been hearing all your life: dress appropriately for the weather; wear practical shoes; stay in safe, well-traveled areas; drink plenty of water; and keep your eye out for anyone who makes you uncomfortable. Beyond those basics, though, are a few others that are worth your consideration:

- Choose your route wisely. Always know exactly where your walking route will take you, and have an idea of how long you expect to be gone. If you're not certain a particular street or field or park is a safe place to walk with your dog, drive or bike the route first at the time of day you intend to walk to see if you'll feel comfortable. Always try out any new route during daylight hours.

  In addition to scoping out your routes in advance, let a friend, neighbor, or family member know what routes you typically take and the time frame of your walks. Always carry some form of identification. If you have a cell phone, bring it along for use in any emergency.

- Mind the traffic. Whenever possible, choose routes that keep both you and your dog away from speeding cars. When you must walk along a busy road, walk facing traffic, with your dog to your left, away from the road. Your dog is both less intelligent about how people drive and less visible to drivers than you are and needs the extra distance to keep him safe. If you live in a city, make a habit of crossing at crosswalks.

HEALTHY ALTERNATIVES TO JUNK-FOOD FOR YOU AND YOUR DOG

We know every person's tastes are different (and for that matter, so are every dog's), but we're sure even the pickiest eater can find something to enjoy on these lists of healthful snacks for people and for dogs. Whatever snack you choose, read labels to be sure you understand how much makes a serving size—even the healthiest of choices isn't going to help in your weight-loss program if it's being eaten in bulk!

BETTER GOODIES FOR PEOPLE

- *Any* fresh fruit or vegetable
- Baked chips
- Salsa instead of any sauce or dip
- Jell-O Fat Free Pudding Snacks
- Quaker Low-Fat Granola Bars
- Pretzel rods
- Low-fat popcorn
- Welch's Fruit Juice Bars
- Fat-Free Fudgsicle
- Flavored rice cakes
- Angel food cake
- Whole-grain crackers
- Low-fat yogurt
- Light string cheese

BETTER GOODIES FOR DOGS

- Baby carrots
- Frozen green beans, frozen peas, or frozen diced carrots
- Blueberries (frozen or fresh)
- Small shredded wheat squares
- Cheerios

- Training-size treats (these tiny treats are often made of freeze-dried liver or dehydrated fish/beef/poultry and are available in pet-supply stores and department and grocery stores with big pet-supply sections)
- Apple slices
- Flavored rice cakes (broken in pieces)

- Be prepared for your specific health issues. If you have a special health concern, set yourself up for success by being ready to handle problems that could come up during a walk. For example, if you have diabetes or another blood-sugar imbalance, carry a small snack. If you suffer from severe allergies, carry a treatment when you walk. If you have asthma, bring along an inhaler. Everyone should bring water for any walk longer than twenty minutes or so.

7. Be Prepared to Protect Your Dog Along the Way

WHILE many of the safe walking concerns for dogs are the same as they are for people, there are a few that are more uniquely canine:

- Stop at all curbs. A good rule of paw to follow while leash-walking your city dog is to make him stop and sit at every curb and wait for permission to cross the street. This is sometimes hard for the human to remember, so you decide if this will be a rule or not. It might save your dog's life in the future. Here's how to do it. Begin with a dog that already knows the SIT command. When you get to the curb, politely

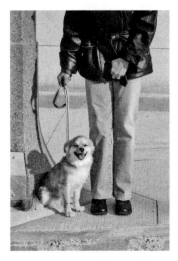

request a SIT, and just stand there until you get the SIT. If the dog is confused, it is okay to guide him into the SIT, but you must insist on a SIT before crossing the street. No scolding is allowed, since it ruins the fun. The dog will quickly learn that sitting is the quickest way to move things forward. If your city has no curb, then try to enforce this before crossing any street, even without the curb. This good walking habit not only might prevent a loose dog from crossing a street, but is also an opportunity to practice the SIT command. Remember to praise each and every SIT. The dog's real reward will be continuing the walk.

● Mind the cold a little. Odds are that your dog can tolerate cold temperatures as well or better than you can. A chill in the air will seldom bother any dog with a full coat. In cases of extreme cold, thin dogs, short-haired dogs, and senior pets can benefit from having their own coat or sweater. (A dog jacket will keep road salt from irritating the skin on your dog's belly, too.) If you decide to buy one, choose something waterproof and easy to clean. As great as that little white wool number looks on Rover in the pet-superstore aisle, it won't hold up to even one long winter walk and the sludge that comes with it. Dr. Becker's dogs use snazzy Lycra bodysuits that stretch, breathe, keep them warm, protect from snow, ice, and salt, and go straight into the washing machine. For more information, check out www.k9topcoat.com.

Coats may be optional for dogs, but boots are essential. They'll keep salt, ice chips, and mud from melting snow from getting between your dog's paw pads. At the least, boots will help keep your floors clean (and take away "the mess it makes" as a reason for not walking!), but more importantly, they'll prevent skin irritations and infections on your dog's

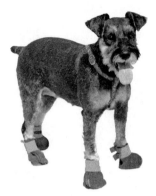

sensitive paws. Boots, like collars, take a bit of getting used to for dogs, but the adjustment period should be handled the same way as for a new collar or leash (page 119): put the boots on your dog, give him a nice treat, then ignore him while he gets adjusted to the joys of fancy footwear.

On the bright side, as long as he's got his boots on (and maybe the stretchy suit that makes him look like a four-footed speed skater), odds are there will never be a day when the weather is warm enough for you but too cold for your workout buddy.

● Mind the heat a lot. Even though your dog tolerates cold better than you, he's ill equipped to deal with high heat. Humans and dogs both evaporate water to cool their bodies. Whereas humans sweat over the entire surface of their bodies, dogs sweat only a little bit from the pads of their feet and primarily through the evaporative surface of their tongue. Factor in a full-length fur coat and (in the case of many dogs) a substantial layer of insulating fat, and you're dealing with an animal who can very quickly overheat and become very sick because of it.

Seven considerations come into play when you decide whether, when, and where to walk your dog in hot weather:

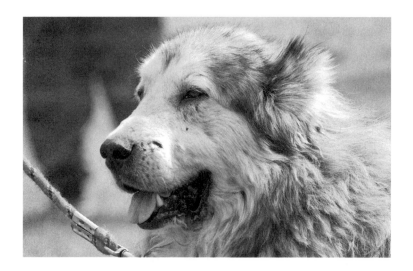

1. **What is his body size?** Larger dogs are at increased risk of overheating because the evaporative surface-to-volume ratio goes down with increasing size. For example a Great Dane (thirty inches high) doesn't have a much bigger tongue than a Welsh corgi (ten to twelve inches high).

2. **What is his body accustomed to?** A dog who lives and walks daily in Texas is going to fare far better on a ninety-degree day than one who walks in Vermont and rarely experiences such high temperatures. If you're dealing with an unseasonably hot day, consider walking your dog on a shorter route, choosing shade, and frequently offering water.

3. **What is the level of humidity?** A hot day is hard on any dog, but a hot, humid day does even more to curb his ability to cool off.

4. **On what surface will your dog be treading?** The risk of heat exhaustion or more serious heat complications is often paired

with the risk of scalded paws from hot pavement. If you're thinking of walking on a hot, sunny day, test the pavement surface with the palm of your hand before expecting your dog to follow along. If the ground is too hot for your hand, it's dangerous for your pooch's feet, so choose either a different time or a route with grass and/or dirt surfaces instead.

5. **When can we catch a heat break?** Success in any exercise program means sticking to it, so the last thing we want you to do is forego your walks with your dogs for June, July, and August. Instead, try to schedule them before 10 a.m. or after 7 p.m., when the temperature will be more manageable.

6. **Water your dog, inside and out.** There's just no substitute for the handy-dandy squirt bottle. Bring along a full one—or some other source of water—for every warm-weather walk with your dog. Use your dog's water to "hose" him down periodically, and to make sure he has frequent opportunity to drink. We know several walkers who fill up a special backpack designed to hold water for hikers and campers (available at department stores like Wal-Mart) and use that to keep their dogs hydrated on hot days.

7. **Know what to do if heatstroke happens.** Signs of heatstroke in your dog can include exhaustion, staggering or a lack of coordination, vomiting or labored breathing, and panting. If you suspect your dog has hyperthermia or heatstroke, call an emergency veterinarian immediately. Taking the dog's temperature will provide valuable information for the veterinarian. (This can be done rectally or with an ear thermometer. We recommend the Pet-Temp Instant Ear Thermometer because it is reasonably priced and accurate. For more information, visit www.pet-

WHILE WE'RE ON THE SUBJECT OF WATER . . .

Keeping yourself hydrated is just as important as doing so for your dog. Not drinking enough prevents you from walking to the best of your ability. Don't wait until you're thirsty to have water, because by then your body is desperate for it. Instead, stick to the following plan:

- Drink one 8-ounce glass of water two hours before exercise.
- Drink an 8-ounce glass of water ten minutes before exercise.
- Drink at least one 8-ounce glass of water after exercise.

temp.com.) Dogs' normal temperatures generally range between 101 and 103. A temperature of 104 or higher requires an effort to cool the dog down. A temperature of 106 should be considered an extreme emergency and treated by a veterinarian.

Cool your dog by gentle hosing with cool water or immersing for a short time (no more than fifteen minutes) in cool water (don't let his head get in the water). Wet his fur and blow air over him with a fan. Use cool or tepid water, not ice-cold water, as it's possible to overcool your dog and make the situation worse.

A case of "heat stress" in a dog may resolve on its own, once you help him cool down. But a moderate to severe case—if your dog is exhibiting abnormal symptoms like being unsteady on his feet or unconscious, vomiting, or having seizures—will require the services of a veterinarian.

8. Know When to Quit

DOGS love to walk and they love to run. While some are reasonably smart about knowing when to stop and rest a bit, many are not. We have seen dogs walk, run, or chase tennis balls until they literally collapse from exhaustion. If your dog is not the kind to sit down and quit when he's had enough, you'll need to pay close attention to reading the signs that he's tired:

- If your dog customarily wants to lead the way (or heels beautifully), he may need a break if he starts lagging behind you on a walk.
- If he's breathing heavily with his tongue hanging, it's time for a break.
- If your dog's gait becomes clumsy or looks awkward or unusual to you, stop for a while.
- If your dog tries to stop, sit down, or lie down late in a walk, let him rest a minute before moving on.

Now that you've waded through all the cautions and preparations, we'd like to remind you of the health benefits you stand to reap from starting and sticking to this program. Research has demonstrated that the benefits of walking can include, among other things, weight loss, increased muscle mass, protection against heart disease, reduced cholesterol levels, improved bone density, increased self-esteem, and decreased depression.

If you're ready to start feeling those benefits for yourself (and seeing how walking tremendously benefits your dog), lace up your walking shoes and follow the instructions in the coming pages.

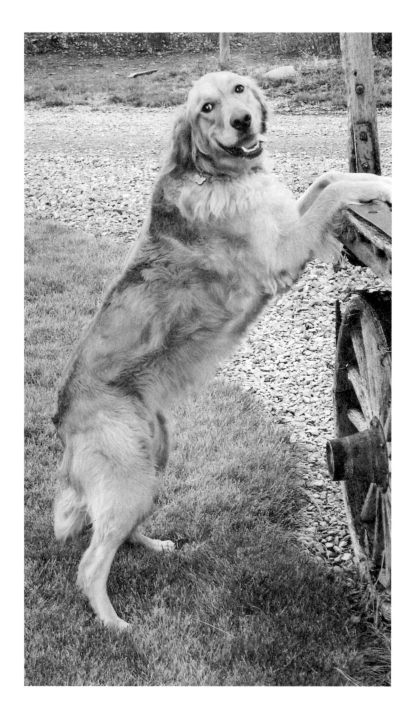

CHAPTER 6

Let the Workouts Begin

Do you know the cost of taking off a pound? It's about 3,500 calories, either cut by eating less or burned off in exercise. And gosh yes, that does sound like a lot.

The commitment to starting (and sticking to) an exercise routine and tackling all those calories can certainly seem daunting. We have found (as have many researchers who study the science of weight loss) that the key to success is finding a program that suits your personality and gels with your lifestyle—then sticking to it. Having the ability to truly improve your dog's health, happiness, and longevity is one powerful motivator. That motivation is the reason that when the participants in the PPET study showed up week after week at the Wellness Institute, not just following the instructions for eating better and exercising with their dogs, but also happy and enthusiastic to be spending regular workout time with their furry best friends, we knew we needed to sit up and take notice. After all, if you're walking lots and eating wisely, and if you're enjoying yourself all the while, burning off 3,500 extra calories in a week is a very achievable goal.

In this chapter, we'll show you how to boost your metabolism and senses. If you stick with your new routine, you'll melt away your own excess pounds and the ones on your dog, by tackling them literally step by step, one teeny-tiny calorie at a time.

Where Do We Start?

FITNESS Unleashed is divided into two levels, and deciding which one to begin with is simply a matter of discovering the lowest common exercise denominator for you and your dog. If either of you is an exercise novice, start at the first level and work your way up. Whether you're a lifetime runner and your dog is an overweight couch potato or you're the sofa spud and the dog is the sprinter in the family, it's important to give the participant who has the least experience with exercise a chance to ease into the program and build up some stamina before progressing to the next level.

Six Steps to Ensure Success

1. STICK TO IT!

This should really be numbers 1, 2, and 3, because it's *that* important. Follow the four-week plans and then choose the level of activity you're comfortable maintaining week after week. If you lose a week along the way, start again where you left off—and act like Velcro and keep sticking.

THE RIGHT START

If you tested as a Doggie Doorkeeper . . .

Start at Level One, regardless of your dog's results.

If you tested as a Stop-and-Go Stroller . . .

Start at Level One, regardless of your dog's results.

If your dog tested as a Passive Pooch . . .

Start at Level One, regardless of your own results.

If your dog tested as a Fragile Fido . . .

Start at Level One, regardless of your own results.

If you tested as a Same-Route Repeater and your dog is a Good Buddy or an Energizer Pup . . .

Start at Level Two.

If you tested as a Fur-Free Fitness Fan and your dog is a Good Buddy or an Energizer Pup . . .

Start at Level Two.

2. HELP YOUR DOG HELP YOU

The best way to bring your dog on board as a full participant in your exercise program is to walk at the same time every day you go. "Dogs have excellent biological clocks," explains Dr. Rolan Tripp, the veterinarian in La Mirada, California. "If you make anything a pattern in their lives, they'll start looking to it and waiting for it. In short, if you keep your exercise routine to a regular time of day, your four-footed 'exercise machine' will not only go along with you—he will seek you out and remind you."

In short, the best time for a workout is the one that'll be the easiest for you to stick to—whether it's first thing in the morning, after dinner at night, or anytime in between. Your dog will be best able to help you stick to it if your routine falls not only at close to the same time, but also at the same juncture in your routine (for example: right after your morning coffee). We know a Labrador retriever named Francine who gets her walk every night after her owner puts the family's three children to bed. Francine stretches out on the floor and snores in the children's rooms while they get ready for bed, hear

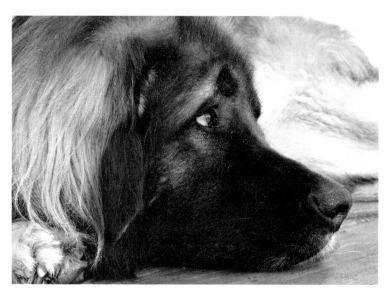

their stories, and say their prayers, but the minute she hears that third "Amen," she's bouncing off the walls and bounding for the door. There's no doubt in her mind that that magic word means her walk time has finally arrived.

3. WRITE IT DOWN; WRITE IT ALL DOWN

In the appendix of this book you'll find a Fitness Unleashed progress chart that you can either cut out and copy or download from www.diet.com, the online format of Dr. Kushner's Personality Diet weight-loss program. We strongly advise you to post it on your refrigerator, your desk, or your kitchen counter—wherever you'll see it and be reminded to fill it in every single day. The form helps you keep track of your progress, your goals, what you eat, how much you exercise, and how you feel.

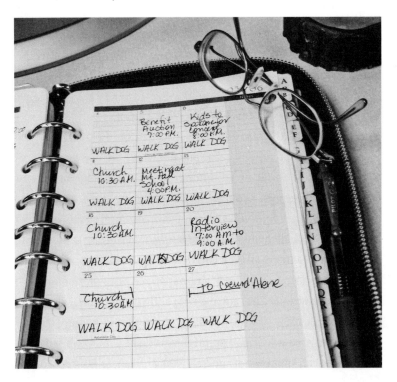

Lest you think keeping track of all this would be a pain in the butt (to keep the pain in your legs company), know that research has shown that people who keep a food and activity diary in conjunction with a weight-loss program have a 25 percent higher success rate than those who don't.

4. FEEL THAT SWEET E-MOTION

If you or your dog is feeling tired, discouraged, or depressed (and yes, dogs definitely do sometimes feel depressed), Judith Shoemaker, DVM, a complementary veterinary medicine and therapy practitioner and educator, explains that there's really nothing quite like a walk to give you a psychological boost. "It's very hard to be down when you're sticking your chest out with your head held high," she explains. "Your emotion takes over and it makes you feel active and positive."

So, when the prospect of burning calories isn't motivation enough to help you get up and get moving, do it for the positive energy burst instead.

5. BE READY WITH BAD-WEATHER PLANS

Into every life, a little rain and snow must fall. So the question is, do you have boots and an umbrella? Since walking the dog is traditionally (and most enjoyably) an outdoor activity, a change of seasons can really shake up your routine. Typically, spring and fall are "walkable" everywhere, while folks in some climates find brutal summer heat the most challenging and others have a hard time dealing with frigid, snowy winters. If you're not willing or able to walk in all weather, you need to have your alternative activities plotted out.

In most communities, anyone who really wants to walk can find an indoor location. If you doubt it, clip on your pedometer and check it out. A couple trips around the inside of a mall (walking, not shopping!) can quickly add up to 1,000 or even 2,000 steps. Many

THE DREADED SCALE

No, nobody wants to stand on it, but the scale gives you a down-and-dirty assessment of your progress and it's an important part of tracking the effectiveness of your routine. We do not recommend weighing yourself every day. Instead, plan on weighing yourself once a week, at the same time of day, and always on the same scale. This will give you a fairly objective measure of your success. Keep in mind that it may take several days or even longer to see a difference in this least forgiving of self-assessments. During that time, stay positive by focusing on other measures of success, like the increased energy level that comes from sticking to a walking routine and the likely development that your clothes will feel more comfortable before the scale can calculate any progress.

You can also track your dog's progress with regular (though perhaps less frequent) weigh-ins. Most veterinary offices are happy to let their clients stop by to weigh their dogs on a weekly, biweekly, or monthly basis to monitor weight loss.

churches, community centers, and colleges have indoor walking tracks that are available to the public. Unfortunately, most of these alternative walking destinations are not dog friendly (big sigh). With that in mind, you'll need to make up the exercise for Fido, too. Luckily many cities are developing four-season dog parks where the fur can fly. And don't forget: pet megastores welcome four-legged shoppers, so you and your dog can walk there, too.

If your dog is among the many breeds who are ball or Frisbee crazy, you've got a guaranteed fast workout for him, even if you have to stand under an umbrella to get it in. If he's not a ball chaser, try enlisting a friend or family member to get him to play "tag" or "hide-

and-seek" at home. To do this, split up inside and take turns calling him to you and offering a small treat for his trouble. If you've got kids, encourage them to enlist the dog in an active, indoor game, such as tossing a toy down the hallway for him to retrieve "rover and rover" again. While none of these is a long-term substitute for a regular walk, all of them give a dog the opportunity to run, stretch, and burn calories at home.

If you want to get your exercise at home and you have a staircase, you're in luck. Researchers have found that climbing steps for fifteen minutes burns a comparable number of calories to walking for thirty. Your dog can climb the staircase with you. To motivate him (because we know a lot of dogs who will opt not to climb stairs once they see you're doing it for no apparent good reason), toss a small treat to the top of the stairwell as you embark on each "lap" and then stand back—you wouldn't want to trip over that speeding bundle of hungry dog while you're climbing, right?

Lastly, if you're just going to go for your walk despite the weather (remember that, like the famed slogan for the U.S. Postal Service, nothing will keep dogs from their appointed rounds), review the

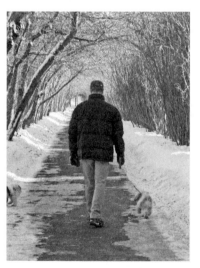

weather-safety guidelines in Chapter 5 and outfit yourself and your dog appropriately. Keep in mind that simple route choices can substantially mitigate weather problems. Choosing a shady path on a hot day will help keep you and your dog cool, for example. Choosing a nonpaved path on a snowy day will reduce your chances of slipping and sliding on ice.

6. FOR MAXIMUM IMPACT, CHOOSE DIET CHANGES, TOO.

There is no question that undertaking the exercise portion of this program—even if you don't make changes in your diet—will improve your level of fitness. There is also no question that if you want to lose weight, you'll be able to do so significantly more quickly if you also follow the diet and nutrition recommendations for your eating personality in Chapter 3. You don't have to severely restrict your diet to lose weight with Fitness Unleashed, but by eating fewer unhealthy snacks and more fruits and vegetables, and paying attention to portion sizes, you'll see better results, and see them sooner.

Starter Week for Levels One and Two

WHETHER you're entering this program at Level One or Level Two, follow these simple Week One instructions to get on the right track.

Step right. The most effective and safest walking technique is one in which your posture is tall and your back is straight. Your feet should swing through with the heel striking first and rolling to the ball of the foot with each step. Anytime you decide to pick up the pace, do so by taking more steps of the same length, rather than by lengthening or shortening your step. Taking more steps with your normal gait will burn more calories than longer steps, and it will help prevent injuries that can be caused by overstretching with an overly long stride.

In Level One, simply choose the gait that is most comfortable for you and let your arms swing naturally. Later in this chapter, we'll explain how you can incorporate some upper-body work in your regular routine, too.

When it comes down to it, much of the effectiveness of your routine will be determined by the pace at which you choose to walk. If you're new to exercise, please take your time working up to speed. For regular walkers and those later in the program, the ideal pace should feel something like the one you'd use if you were late for a bus or a train—hustling, but not frantic. If you're walking at a window-shopping pace, you're only going to begin to tap the benefits of Fitness Unleashed.

Post your Eating and Activity Log. Put your log in a spot where you'll see it and remember to fill it in. We truly can't overestimate the value of filling out one of these forms every week. It allows you to literally "see the big picture" of your efforts, and it'll encourage you to build on your own progress each week. You'll find a template in the Appendix at the back of the book. If you prefer, you can print blank copies of the form from www.diet.com. Plan to post a new form on the same day each week. Keep your forms from previous weeks so you can see how you're improving over time.

Choose your food goals for this week. Review the recommended changes for your eating pattern in Chapter 3, then choose two diet mini-goals from the list in this chapter (see page 156) to undertake this week. Pick only two, and note them at the top of your log sheet. Sample mini-goals for this week: Eat a fruit or vegetable with every meal. Give your dog two vegetable snacks this week.

Commit to your dog's new diet. We all know that changing our own diets is more difficult than changing a dog's—after all, most dogs eat only what they're given, while we have to make our own choices from meal to meal and day to day. While your transition to a healthy, satisfying diet that allows weight loss may take some time and trial and error, you can start measuring and feeding your dog according to the veterinarian's recommendations today. This week, put the measuring cup with the food and use it every time you dish out a meal.

Start stretching. Gentle stretching is the best starting point for any exercise routine. It'll help prevent injuries during your walks, increase your range of motion, release tension, and wake up your muscles. Before each stretching session, walk five minutes at a comfortable pace (or march in place) to warm up your muscles. As you stretch, breathe naturally. Don't bounce or overstretch to the point of pain. Repeat each stretch twice. Whenever possible, do the following four stretches before each walk:

● Reach for the sky: Stretch your arms above your head and extend your fingers to their full reach. Now turn your hands palms-up and interlock your fingers. Hold for 15 seconds.

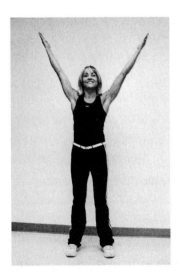 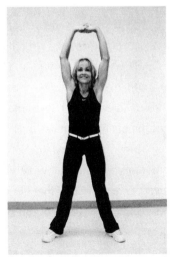

THE VETERINARIAN SAYS: DOES FIDO NEED TO STRETCH?

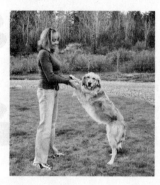

You may be wondering if your dog requires stretching as part of Fitness Unleashed. The simple answer is no. If you observe him carefully, you'll find he probably does plenty of stretching on his own—especially the big, long, back-arching ones when he first wakes in the morning and after naps.

But could your dog benefit from stretching, and might he love having you help him with it? Well, that's a yes.

Every morning, my wife, Teresa, stretches our beloved mix-breed bed hog Quixote. She holds him by the back legs and gently pulls them straight out behind him, and Quixote, who clearly knows his part of this exercise, extends and contracts his front toes rhythmically, like a cat clawing for traction, as he bends his back. You can easily see the muscles tighten and then loosen all along the length of his body. Sometimes, we stretch him together. Teresa takes his front legs and I grab his back legs and we say, "Okay, let's make a taffy-dog," and give him a gentle stretch. Quixote *loves* this. He loves the hands-on attention; he loves the feeling of the stretch itself; and he loves the big fuss we make over him. He wiggles with joy every time.

My friend and colleague Narda Robinson, DVM, an expert in complementary and alternative veterinary medicine at Colorado State University, emphasizes that pet owners who wish to stretch their dogs should be looking for the kind of reaction we get from Quixote—a happy-dog response. "Most of the dogs I treat have tension in their backs or legs that massage and stretching might ease," she explains, "and if your dog enjoys the experience, it can be beneficial." But if your dog seems uncomfortable, tense, or just not content with stretching, then consider this a job he does best by himself.

Stretch your calves: Stand with your hands at your hips and one foot several inches forward. Bend your front leg to stretch the calf muscle of your rear leg, keeping both heels flat on the ground and all ten toes pointing forward. Hold for 15 seconds, then switch legs.

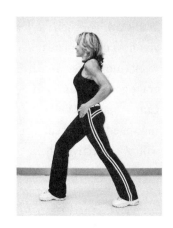

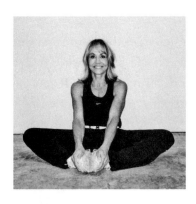

Sitting stretch: To stretch the groin muscles before a walk, sit on the floor with the soles of your feet touching each other and hold your toes with your hands. Bend forward at the hips as far as you are comfortable and hold for 15 seconds.

Hamstring stretch: Sit with one leg bent and the other leg stretched out straight at a 45-degree angle to the side. Bend forward at your hips, leaning toward and facing the straight leg, and keep your head upright. Hold for 15 seconds and repeat for both legs.

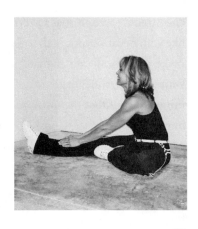

Walk on. For each week and each level of Fitness Unleashed, we tell you how to calculate the number of steps to add to your routine that week (most often 10 percent). However, we've also calculated an average goal for our math-averse participants and labeled it the Cookie Cutter option. While this version of the program is not as carefully calibrated to your current level of fitness as the step-count version, it will still effectively help you build up the frequency, duration, and intensity of your walks.

Level One Four-Week Start

IF either you or your dog is new to exercise, this is your starting place. This four-week program ensures a safe, steady switch from a sedentary lifestyle to a more active one for both of you. If your responses to our exercise-patterns quiz put you in the Doggie Doorkeeper or Stop-and-Go Stroller categories, there's a good chance both you and your dog are leading a less active lifestyle and could immensely—and almost immediately—benefit from Fitness Unleashed. If you're starting from square one, you may think losing weight and getting fit will be too much hard work, but we've got good news for you: over the years, some of the most remarkable and encouraging weight-loss results we've seen have been for beginners like you. Because your activity level is very low, you'll find that if you make only moderate changes in your diet and add short walks to your routine, you'll begin to see results. And if you're overweight, remind yourself that the more a person weighs, the more calories they burn during exercise. Consider it Mother Nature's way of giving you a boost ahead in your quest for weight loss.

FITTING IN FITNESS

As you gradually raise your daily step count, your goal should be to raise your dog's daily step count, too. When you walk together consistently, that's bound to happen. However, don't limit your extra steps to the ones you're taking with your dog. Squeeze them in wherever you can. Try any one, or two, or ten of the following suggestions for working extra steps into an average day to see which ones work for you. You may be surprised when you check your pedometer to see how big a difference these little changes can make:

- Take the stairs instead of the elevator.
- Get off your bus or train one stop early and walk.
- Pace your office, your house, or your yard while you talk on a cordless phone.
- Walk to a coworker's office instead of e-mailing.
- Take a walk while waiting for an appointment.
- Walk once around the mall (or even a big department store) before you shop.
- Walk your child to school.
- Work in your garden or yard (raking, weeding, shoveling snow, and mowing the lawn—with a push mower—are all great exercise).
- Have your morning coffee during a stroll around the block.
- When unloading groceries from the car, carry them inside one bag at a time.
- Take a 10-minute walk before eating lunch.
- Carry laundry through your home one small pile at a time.
- Play hide-and-seek or tag or kickball with your kids (or your grandkids, or your neighbor's kids).

WEEK 1

Walk this way! In addition to following the Starter Week instructions (page 141), look at the three-day pedometer average you created in Chapter 5, then add 10 percent to that number. (For example, if your average was 3,000 steps, this week you'll strive to average 3,300 steps per day. If your average was 5,000 steps, make it 5,500.) That's your step target for each day this week. So that you and your dog can both start benefiting right away, we want you to take those extra steps together whenever you can. Wear your pedometer on your walks to be sure you're actually getting as many steps as you intend. Write down your step total every night so you can calculate a new average at the end of the week.

Continue to stretch before every walk. When you reach the point where you are breaking a sweat during your walks, it's also time to add a 5-minute slow-paced cool-down walk as part of your routine.

Cookie Cutter Option: The Level One, Week 1 Cookie Cutter goal is three to four walks of at least 15 minutes each. (Note: Keep your pedometer on if you choose this option—you'll still need an average of your steps this week to make sure you're making progress in subsequent weeks.)

Choose your mini-goals. *Sample mini-goals for this week: Keep meal-replacement bars at home for grab-and-go breakfasts. Choose a fresh fruit instead of one sweet treat.*

WEEK 2

First things first—post your paperwork. Add up your step counts from Week 1 and divide by seven to get your new average. Fill in your step count on this week's new Eating and Activity Log and post it where you'll remember to keep filling it out every day. Even though you're taking deliberate walks for exercise only three or four days a week at this point, your long-term goal is to raise your step

TURN AROUND!

Starting at the end of this week, provided your balance is not impaired, we'd like you to turn around and walk 25 steps backward, two separate times, on each walk you take. Walking backward challenges your coordination, it works your leg muscles in different places than forward walking, and it challenges your dog to keep his eye on you at all times, lest you should suddenly decide to change direction. Walking backward burns substantially more calories than walking forward, but its purpose here is most importantly to awaken a different portion of your musculature.

count for every day, and keeping track will help you measure your progress toward that goal. We often find that patients who wear pedometers and begin adding steps while walking a few days per week also soon start adding steps on their "off" days as well!

Choose your weekly food goals. Choose two mini-goals for this week—and make sure at least one of them is a new one. If you'd like to carry over one or both of last week's goals, good for you, but do add at least one goal that's new. *Sample mini-goals: Split an entrée at a restaurant. Compare food labels and choose one healthier alternative to your usual food.*

Stretch before every walk. See pages 143–145 for information on stretching.

Add another 10 percent. Using your newly calculated step average from last week, add another 10 percent and make this your goal

ALL ABOUT HEART RATE

Knowing your heart rate will help you better assess the intensity of your walking regimen. First, to figure out your maximal heart rate, just subtract your age from 220. (For example, say you're forty; 220 − 40 = 180—and that's your maximal rate.) Now, to calculate your actual heart rate, gently rest the pads of your middle and index fingers against your neck beneath your jawline. Once you've located the rhythm of your heartbeat, count how many beats you feel over a period of six seconds. Add a zero to that number and you've got your heart rate. If you're new to exercise, your goal during a walk should be to achieve a heart rate of about 60 percent of your maximal rate (in the case of the forty-year-old mentioned above, that will be 108 beats per minute or so). As you become more fit, you'll be able to work at a higher level of intensity and get that heart rate higher, up into the 75 percent range.

for a daily average this week. Take a good chunk of these steps over the course of four walks this week. **Cookie Cutter Option:** This week, take at least four walks of at least 20 minutes each. Wear that pedometer!

WEEK 3
Look at that step count! If you have successfully upped your step count by 10 percent for two consecutive weeks, you'll see a significant jump in that number from Week 1 when you post your Eating and Activity Log this week. Congratulations on the progress you've

already made. If you've been minding your eating-personality advice from Chapter 4, by now you're losing between a half a pound and a pound a week. It's a slow start, but you should also be feeling more energy and stamina this week—and, *so*, it's time to up your walking goal again!

Add another 10 percent. By now, this math is getting easy for you, though adding each 10 percent on top of your step count should be getting a little more challenging. This week's **Cookie Cutter Option** is at least four walks of at least 25 minutes each.

Do your stretches before every walk. And take a few minutes to cool down after.

Start experimenting with intensity. In the second level of the program, intensity is the name of the game. At this point, though, it's time to give your body a feel for your range of speeds and levels of effort. On one walk this week, divide your 25 minutes as follows: 10 minutes at your usual pace, then 5 minutes at a faster pace than you're accustomed to. (If you think you're working too hard after 5 minutes, test yourself by trying to speak a sentence without gasping for air. If you can't, take a minute to catch your breath before moving on.) If you can speak without gasping, take your heart rate (instructions on page 150) as you slow your pace and continue with another 10 minutes of regular-paced walking.

Choose your eating goals. You can choose to continue up to two of the goals you've already undertaken, but add at least one that's new. *Sample mini-goals for this week: Order a dressing or sauce on the side. Cook with olive oil instead of butter. Prepare an entrée with twice the veggies and half the meat the recipe calls for.*

WALKING SAVES A LIFE

If you think your dog is too young, old, small, or sickly to take on a walking routine, we'd love for you to talk with our friend Dr. Veronika Kiklevich, a veterinarian in San Antonio, Texas, and coauthor of *Real People Don't Own Monkeys*. Dr. Kiklevich readily admits she became a veterinarian so she could indulge her love of animals, and that her role in doing so over the years—in addition to treating her patients—has included bringing home all sorts of pets that were labeled hopeless cases. Because of her strong conviction that exercise is key to good health, this veterinarian has put dogs of all breeds on walking programs, including a few who were one step away from euthanasia because of their health problems.

One of those dogs is Oso, a Labrador retriever who was brought to the veterinary office as a puppy. "His owner brought him in thinking he had a neurological problem because of his very painful, awkward gait," Dr. Kiklevich explains, "but I thought the problem might be orthopedic, and I had him radiographed. Even at that young age, his hips were fairly tragic. The problem was terrible hip dysplasia," a condition in which the hip socket no longer works like a perfect ball-and-socket joint but becomes unstable and painful.

The orthopedic specialist who saw Oso recommended that the owner have him euthanized, but Dr. Kiklevich delivered the news with an option. "I told the owner I'd take Oso, that I'd have his hips replaced if it needed to be done, and that I'd put him down if I had to rather than make him suffer."

Then the veterinarian took Oso home to her family and put him on a gentle exercise program, starting with short walks and working up to longer ones, always paying attention to whether Oso seemed uncomfortable or as if he'd had enough.

At this writing, Oso is healthy, happy, and a canine senior citizen at eleven years old. Even though Dr. Kiklevich has faithfully had Oso's hips checked every six months since he was a puppy, Oso never had to have them replaced.

"I kept asking if he needed to have the hip replacement," Dr. Kiklevich explains, "but the orthopedic experts were amazed at how well he was doing." She attributes much of Oso's nearly miraculous change of health to the long, slow walks he's had all his life. Over the years, Dr. Kiklevich says his amazing turnaround has been an inspiration to the owners of other pets she treats (including a few cats!) to get their own four-legged friends out and exercising, too.

WEEK 4

Wow, what a good-looking dog you've got there. If you started feeding your dog according to the veterinarian's recommendations in Week 1, and if you've kept up with your walking routine thus far, we're willing to bet that by now you're seeing a difference in your dog. Odds are he's lost a pound and maybe more. Is he chomping at the bit at walk time every day? Is he sleeping better, longer? Is he rising more easily and does he have a kick in his step getting up the stairs? If so, congratulations! You have officially made significant strides toward improving your dog's health and lengthening his life. He may not know enough to say "thank you," but we do.

If your dog is not beginning to look and feel more fit, or if he's the rare pooch who's still not finding much joy in walking, turn to Chapter 7, "Making It Fun for Fido," for tips on how to help him not only participate in but also enjoy and benefit from the program.

Tack on another 10 percent. If you started this program at 3,000 steps a day, you should be up to almost 4,500 steps by now. If you started at 4,000, you're approaching 6,000. And if you came in at 5,000, you're closing in on 7,500 steps a day this week. Though everyone walks at a unique pace, the average increase in daily distance covered for those ranges is a little more or less than a mile a day. **Cookie Cutter Option:** Add 5 minutes to each walk this week, making your total four walks of 30 minutes each.

Keep stretching. Now that you've been stretching and walking for three weeks, you're developing a sense of what kinds of exercise really feel good for your body. For many people, one of the highlights is stretching, and those drawn to this kind of exercise supplement their walking workouts with a stretching, yoga, tai chi, or Pilates class or videotape. You can borrow a tape from a friend or the library and give it a try this week, or find a class that works with your schedule if you like.

Push past a setback. If you haven't had a week yet when you've blown off your workout or overindulged in a favorite treat, kudos to you. You are in the minority. It is a rare patient, indeed, who undertakes a weight-loss program and never slips up or falls off the program. If you have an off day or even two this week, we want you to choose to dwell on what you *have* done right on the program so far and what you intend to do right on it in the immediate future. Choose one exercise or mini-goal for today and stick to it. Choose another one tomorrow. By continuing to make small choices that you know are good for you, you'll be 100 percent back on track.

Choose your eating goals. Choose at least two goals this week. *Sample mini-goals: Choose a healthy preportioned meal instead of a self serve–style one. Drink 64 ounces of water every day this week. Make a chopped salad with a variety of fresh vegetables.*

As you reach the end of Level One, it's time to make an informed decision. If you feel you're making steady progress toward your weight and fitness goals on the Level One program, you may want to stay here at the Week 4 level for a while. If you're feeling great and want to push yourself harder, or if your scale is telling you you need more of a workout to really make a difference, it's time to step up to Level Two.

Level Two

WEEK 1
Add steps, and keep a goal in mind. If you're starting the program at Level Two, you'll need to follow the Starter Week instructions on page 141, and you'll begin by adding 10 percent to your three-day step-count average from Chapter 5 as your goal for this week. Level One graduates can just add 10 percent to their step-count average from Level One, Week 4. No matter which group you're in, strive to include your dog as you take many of those extra steps this week. (If you're coming up from Level One, you must wonder when all this step adding is going to end. To achieve an optimum amount of exercise, it will someday reach close to 10,000 steps a day. For many of us, this is a lofty, long-term goal, so don't get discouraged if you're still far from it. If you started this program at 2,000 or 3,000 steps and have been gradually, steadily increasing, congratulations on all you've accomplished so far! Keep up the good work and the moderate step increases.) **Cookie Cutter Option:** Instead of adding minutes to each walk this week, consider adding one more walk. If you're starting the program here, this means five walks this week of 30 minutes each.

MINI-GOALS GALORE

- Eat a fruit or veggie with every meal.
- Stock a few meal-replacement bars and preportioned, low-calorie meals.
- Write down every single little thing you eat and take a hard look at the end of the week.
- Split an entrée in a restaurant, or box up half and save it for another night.
- Compare food labels.
- Choose a snack with more fiber, like whole-wheat crackers or a pear.
- Try a soy-based food, such as soy milk or soy nuts.
- Drink 64 ounces (8 glasses) of water each day.
- Choose frozen-fruit Popsicles instead of a higher-fat, higher-calorie sweet snack.
- Order a dressing or sauce on the side and dip your fork in it as you eat instead of pouring it over your food.
- Cook with olive oil instead of butter.
- Halve the oil or butter called for in a stir-fry or casserole or slow-cooker recipe and see if you can tell the difference.
- Spend an hour learning about portion sizes—see what 8 crackers or a $\frac{1}{2}$ cup of ice cream or cereal *really* looks like by counting and measuring your favorite foods.
- Try a vegetable you've never had before.
- Eat a double-the-veggie, half-the-meat entrée.
- Take the stairs—at least two flights.
- Walk a new route—preferably something with a hill!
- Take a walking break instead of a coffee break.
- Measure that dog food!
- Split your dog's daily ration into at least two and up to four servings.

- Don't allow your dog to be present when the family eats (put him outside, in his kennel, or in another room).
- Give your dog tastes of two veggies and see which one he likes best.
- Ditto for fruits.
- If you're going to give other tasty treats to your dog, and you will, use low-calorie ones like freeze-dried liver, chicken, or beef or tiny "training treats" from the pet-food aisle.

Change your route! Both you and your dog will find stimulation and inspiration in a change of scene this week. Consider one of these options:

- Choosing a route that adds some inclines and declines will increase your calories burned and challenge you both.
- Taking a route that has you walking through dirt and grass will work your muscles harder than walking on pavement.
- If you have either option, walking through snow or walking through sand provides a 50 percent or higher boost in calories burned on a walk over a given distance—thus bringing the intensity level of your workout up to something on par with the efforts of a runner.

Choose two eating mini-goals. *Sample mini-goals for this week: Fill your grocery basket without adding anything that's not on your list. Choose a treat of frozen-fruit Popsicles instead of ice cream.*

WEEK 2

Walk faster. Covering more ground in the same amount of time can mean only one thing: more steps and more calories burned. Set your goal this week for a 5 percent increase in your step count, but try to add those steps without significantly adding to your walking time. Now that you've got this thing down, use your time as effectively as possible by picking up the pace to the point where you sweat and start to get winded—though never so much so that you couldn't carry on a conversation. (Not sure? Say something to your dog and see how you do. . . .)

Warm up, stretch out, cool down. As your walks get more athletic, it's time to begin treating yourself more like an athlete—one who needs a warmup and cooldown. Your walk routine should go something like this: 5-minute slow-paced walk to warm up, stretches, increasing intensity/speed-walking period, 5 minutes slow-paced walk to cool down. You might also consider adding a short stretching session after some workouts when your muscles are warm and you're feeling a bit tight.

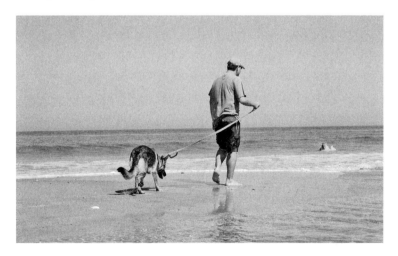

Measure your intensity. Building fitness in the long term requires exercising at a level that challenges your heart, lungs, and entire body. A good way to gauge that level of intensity is to rate the effort or strain you are experiencing while walking. To rate your intensity yourself, use a simple, subjective scale ranging from 0 to 10, where 0 = how you feel at rest and 10 = how you feel if you're working as hard as possible. You want to work at an exertion rating of 6 or 7—a fast pace, but a controlled one. People exercising at this level breathe harder, have an elevated pulse rate, and sweat. All those signs will let you know you're in your target range.

For an alternative measure of intensity, see the information about measuring your heart rate on page 150.

Choose your eating mini-goals. *Sample goals for this week: Treat yourself to a single, measured portion of a food you love and savor it. Eat a fruit or vegetable for an afternoon snack each day.*

WEEK 3
Add another 10 percent to your step count, or add 10 minutes to walks on each of five days. If you're taking the Cookie Cutter Option from Week 1, this will bring you to a level of five walks a week of 40 minutes each.

Use your top half. Oh, that lucky dog! When the two of you go for a walk together, he automatically gets a full-body workout—he's got four on the floor, so to speak, and almost every muscle in his body is working. You, on the other hand, need to make a little extra effort for your arms and upper body, especially considering that for 99 percent of your waking life, your arms are hanging at your sides. Consider these tips:

● Bend your arms at 90-degree angles and pump them from your shoulders as you go. You may even find yourself speeding up as you engage your arms in your walk. Even if you don't, just the simple act of deliberately moving them to keep pace with your legs will help you burn up to 10 percent more calories than just walking alone. To pump your arms while walking your dog, either leave a small amount of slack in the leash or use a retractable leash that's free of any snags and flows freely to and from the receptacle.

● Stay away from weights. Though the idea sounds great, many exercise experts advise against using wrist weights when walking because they can contribute to muscle strains and injuries in the arms, shoulder, neck, and chest. If you enjoy working with weights, try a brief weight routine at the end of your walk—but not during it.

● Try trekking poles for upper-body effect. If you haven't yet seen a walker in your neck of the woods who appears to have lost his or her cross-country skis, we'd like to predict that you will someday soon. A walking trend known as pole walking or Nordic walking is all the rage in Europe and beginning to pop up around the United States. Nordic walking was invented in Finland as a way for skiers to train in the off-season, but has since caught on with the masses. The simple act of carrying and utilizing the poles in a walk engages most of the muscles in your body—up to 95 percent, including many upper body muscles that would otherwise be at rest during a walk.

The question, of course (aside from whether you're self-assured enough to walk with poles in fine weather in the first place), is whether you can do this while walking your dog. Check out the selection of hands-free leashes that attach to a belt around your waist at your local pet-supply store and you'll see that this could be the future of walking for you, too.

WEEK 4

If you've reached this point, congratulations to you! Odds are that, by this time, you've discovered that regular exercise is actually pretty addictive in its own right—not entirely unlike chocolate.

You're currently walking for 40 minutes or more, five times a week. If you stick with that routine, you'll likely continue seeing results for several weeks. But if you want to push forward and do more, you've earned the freedom to be able to pick and choose between some new, more challenging exercise options.

This week, choose one of the following options and replace one walk with it. Replace two walks a week with these exercises in the weeks to come. Because of the relative safety and effectiveness of walking, we don't recommend replacing more than three of your five weekly walks with other activities, unless you're gradually making a transition to jogging. Instead, think of your walking days as a low-impact counterpoint to these high-intensity and sometimes high-impact activities. And as always, make sure both you *and* your dog are equally up to the new challenges. Chances are very good that as your dog has been building up his workout stamina right alongside you, he's in fine form for this phase, too.

No matter which option you choose, continue to begin your workout with a 5-minute walking warmup and your stretches, and utilize a 5-minute cooldown at the end.

Despite the new challenges, this ongoing practice of Fitness Unleashed from here onward is a maintenance program. If you continue to exercise intently for 40 minutes, five times a week, and if you choose healthy foods and eat them in moderation, you should continue to lose weight, gain health, and feel energetic.

40-MINUTE WALK REPLACEMENTS

A longer walk. Let's start with the simple alternative first: How about a 60-minute walk? Or an 80- or 90-minute walk? While it's not practical for most people to set aside that kind of time on a daily basis for a walk routine, many of us can eke it out once (or maybe twice) a week. You might come up with your own version of the "detox walk" that Jane Rudnitsky created for herself and her Labrador retriever at the beginning of Chapter 3: a once- or twice-a-week six-mile route that clears her head and makes her muscles feel great. A long-distance walk offers an excellent aerobic workout for you and your dog.

Hiking. Most of us don't have the good fortune to live within walking distance of a hiking trail, but many are within a short drive of a location with dirt paths and challenging terrain. Take a Saturday morning or a Sunday afternoon and spend it hiking with your dog (and your family, if you like). Negotiating uneven ground and climbing will raise your heart rate and burn as many as double the calories of a "normal" walk. If your hike extends beyond your normal 40-minute walk time, you'll reap even more benefits.

The jogging walk. Ever wonder how a person who routinely walks becomes a person who routinely jogs? Many simply alternate between the two paces, gradually building up stamina to maintain the faster pace for longer periods of time—and eventually for the entire route. Though it's important to note that jogging is harder on knees and joints than walking, you should also know that it burns up to twice as many calories per minute, so it's a great boost to a weight-

RUNNING PAWS

Seth Codosh grew up in Westchester County, New York, running several miles a day with his German shorthaired pointer by his side. Years later, after his career brought him to Manhattan, Codosh would borrow a friend's dog to keep him company on his daily trek. "I really prefer to run with a dog rather than going alone," he explains.

One morning while running through Central Park, Codosh saw a group of dogs on a leisurely stroll with a dog walker and got to thinking about how much those dogs would love the chance to run, too. It was a moment of inspiration, and he almost immediately set about founding Running Paws, a service that gives dogs all over the city the chance to full-out exercise several times a week.

At first, Seth was the only runner, logging as much as twelve miles a day in forty-minute segments with different dogs. He estimates that more than 95 percent of the dogs he "run-tests" to see if they'll do well in the program fit right in. "All dogs run." He smiles. "When I started doing this, I expected to be running Labs and golden retrievers—which I do—but we've also got Chihuahuas and toy poodles who run for a few minutes at a stretch, and Jack Russell terriers who could run forever."

Before long, both clients and runners contacted Seth, hoping to be a part of Running Paws. The runners, many of them students and actors and musicians, wanted part-time jobs and the company of dogs on their runs. The dog owners wanted help exercising their furry best friends—some so they didn't have to deal with exercise-frustration behavior problems, and many because their dogs were overweight and out of shape.

Today, the Running Paws team features twenty runners and hundreds of New York City dogs who are realizing Seth Codosh's vision—having the time of their lives every day and getting their own chance to run.

KNOWING YOUR DOG'S LIMITS

Up until this phase of the program, all the recommended activities and levels of intensity are suitable for almost any healthy dog—with the likely exception of some toy breeds who will not be able to keep up. As long as you make the weather an ongoing consideration (especially when there is a risk of your dog overheating), your dog should be able to work up to and complete the five approximately 40-minute walks we recommend and gain health benefits from doing so.

At this stage of the game, though, as you find ways to further intensify your workouts, dogs tend to diverge into two groups. First, there are those who greet this new level of exertion with a, "Well, it's about time!" attitude. They are truly just beginning to hit their stride as they run alongside a biker or a jogger or leap through the snow while you cross-country ski. Second, there are those who will "top out" at this point and not be able to walk farther, longer, or faster than what they've already mastered. Please pay close attention to your dog's demeanor to be sure you have a handle on which group he belongs to. Dogs who can handle more and more intense activity usually come to it not just willingly, but gleefully. They will consistently demonstrate a desire to keep going. Dogs who are at their limit will be far less enthusiastic, and most notably, they will lag behind. If you are pulling your dog *at all* to keep him exercising with you at this level, he is in over his head. If he is struggling, out of breath, or frequently looking at you with a "Why are you doing this to me?" expression on his face (yes, almost every dog we've ever met has one of these in his repertoire), consider cutting back on your expectations of him.

You can continue to pursue more intense workouts for yourself without sacrificing your dog's opportunities to exercise. Many people we know who are more athletic than their dogs alternate their intense workouts with those that are more dog-friendly, and then incorporate their dogs in the warm-up and cool-down phases on their high-output workout days.

loss program. Be sure to prepare for any jogging effort with a 5- to 10-minute warm-up walk and stretching, and follow it with at least 5 minutes of cool-down time and stretches for your warmed muscles.

In-line skating. Skating burns a comparable number of calories to running or bicycling (far more per minute than walking), but it is easier on your joints. It is also a sport your dog can do with you— but not until you get the hang of it on your own! Be sure to wear the recommended protective equipment and don't go any faster than a pace at which you know you can stop. Once your balance is solid, your dog will love to come along.

Cross-country skiing. Obviously, this isn't a year-round option, but hear us out, because it's definitely a walk replacement worth every minute of your effort. Cross-country skiing rivals walking for its low level of wear and tear on your body, but it burns between two and three times as many calories per minute. If you ski on hilly terrain, it can be even more effective than that—using up to 1,200 calories an hour. Aside from its great caloric consumption, the other beauty of cross-country skiing is that we've rarely met a dog who doesn't find running around outdoors with you on a snowy day to be a true joy. Most dogs don't mind the cold a bit, and yours will also be burning extra fat while he romps through the snow as your companion and guide.

Biking. This option does not always work for both parties, as your dog has to be highly fit and have energy to burn in order to keep up, like the Beckers' dog Shakira, who is the canine equivalent of Lance Armstrong. But biking is excellent, effective exercise for you, burning up to eight hundred calories an hour. For an athletic dog, this can be a great opportunity to get a level of workout you could not otherwise provide. In fact, some sled-dog trainers run their dogs

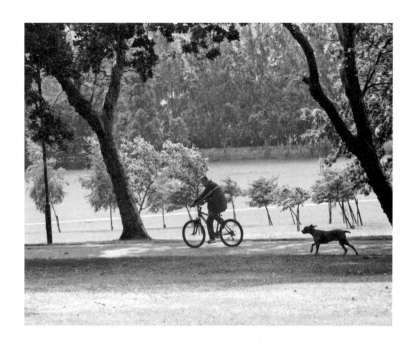

while biking to condition them for the coming winter. A word of caution, though: if you have a dog who is not very strong and fit, ride your bike without him. Because of the intensity of a run-along workout, we strongly recommend you ask your dog's veterinarian for his blessing before you try it with your dog. Always start this program slowly, building up both distance and speed over time. If you do decide to bike with Rover, there are several varieties of bike attachments specially designed to keep your dog beside you and prevent him from upsetting your balance.

ADDING RESISTANCE

As you get accustomed to your walking routine, you may find yourself looking for new challenges and ways to work your muscles. Nothing is a more effective addition to a walking routine than regular, short sessions of resistance training. This kind of muscle-building workout comes in many forms, including calisthenics that utilize your own body mass, weight machines, resistance bands, and free weights. If you are interested in using free weights or resistance bands, we recommend you start out with a resistance-training video or DVD, a class at a local gym, or a consultation with a trainer. Once you've had a chance to experience proper resistance-training technique, you may choose to keep up a routine that includes weights at home.

There are many simple resistance exercises that can be done before, during, or after your walk with your dog to further enhance your program, including the following:

Standing push-ups: Stand facing a wall with your feet a few inches apart and about two feet from the wall. Rest your hands on the wall just below and outside shoulder height and width. Keeping the rest of your body straight, bend your elbows to lower yourself toward the wall and then straighten your elbows to push yourself away from it. Repeat eight to twelve times.

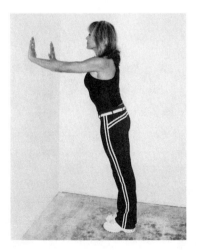
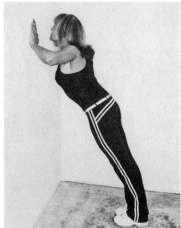

Step-ups: Choose a low bench or a retaining wall that is sturdy enough to support your weight without wobbling or leaning. Place your right leg on this raised surface and use that leg to lift your lower body and left leg up to the same height as the right. Without resting the left foot, lower it back down to the ground with a controlled movement. Repeat eight to twelve times. If you can't do eight repetitions, choose a lower surface. Repeat by placing the left foot on the raised surface and lifting your right side.

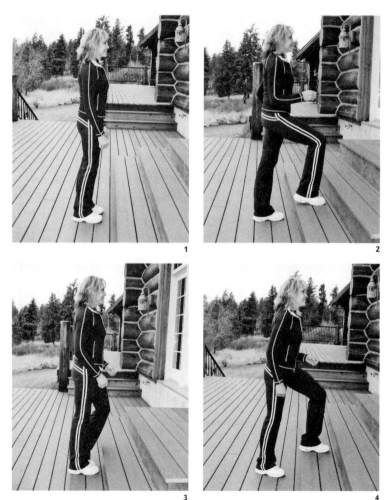

Squats: Stand with your feet shoulder-width apart and rest the palms of your hands on the back of a chair, bench, or other sturdy surface. Keeping your torso straight, slowly bend at the knees and lower yourself until your thighs are parallel to the ground but without your knees going past your toes. Continuing to rely on your leg muscles, slowly raise yourself back to your full height. Repeat eight to twelve times. As your legs strengthen over time, you will no longer need the chair or bench to maintain your balance.

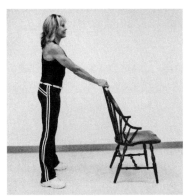 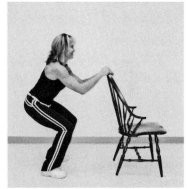

Gym-class classics: All those exercises you did on gym days at school have a respectable role in any health program. At home or at the park, if you can squeeze in eight repetitions each of carefully, slowly executed sit-ups, pull-ups, and lunges every other day, you can expect to steadily gain strength and achieve a higher level of fitness for your time and effort.

The American College of Sports Medicine recommends resistance training for each muscle group no more frequently than every 48 hours. This lag time between workouts gives muscles a chance to rebuild and strengthen after exercise. Of course, you can continue to walk as often as you like.

TREADMILLS FOR TWO

Though it won't give you your daily dose of vitamin D or that wonderful opportunity to connect with the outside world, time on a treadmill is a viable alternative for your regular walk on days when the outside isn't really cooperating. If the weather's getting you down, by all means, steps taken on a treadmill do count.

But what's a dog to do? Just lie around and sullenly watch his best walking buddy work out alone? Turns out, if you're feeling generous (because the upcoming item is quite expensive), your dog can have a treadmill, too.

The Jog-a-Dog exercise treadmill may sound like a silly idea, but we've seen one in action—and seen a dog who had never been on a treadmill immediately take off walking on it—and the machine is pretty darned smart, safe, and well made. These treadmills are often utilized by canine athletes and show dogs, but if you wanted to line one up beside your own, we're sure both you and your four-legged fitness guru would then be able to walk side by side in all weather. More information is available at jogadog.com if you're interested.

CHAPTER 7

Making It Fun for Fido

Let's be honest. Getting a dog to look forward to walking isn't a problem for most pet owners. Typically, the dogs we know are jumping up and down like cheerleaders at walk time, urging, "Okay, let's go! On the floor, out the door, time to go-go-go!" in their language of woofs, wiggles, tail waves, and false starts toward the door. That said, we know that not all dogs are a dream on the end of a leash. As dog owners, we know that a dog's enthusiasm is contagious, and that if your dog is joyful about walking, it'll make it easier for you to find fun in it, too. In this chapter we've assembled ten tips to make your dog a pleasure to walk, and to turn every trip around the park or through your neighborhood into an adventure for both you and your four-legged exercise buddy.

1. The Hansel and Gretel

WHETHER you have a reluctant retriever or an eager beagle, you can foster in your dog a deeply felt love of walking by occasionally seeding his trail with food treats that he can discover and devour. We don't recommend using bread crumbs (remember, the birds ate those in the fairy tale) or putting treats down far in advance (lest the special surprise for *your* dog be gobbled up by someone else's canine connoisseur). Instead, start this walk at a time when your dog is hungry, and with a pocketful of Cheerios, freeze-dried liver morsels, baby carrots, or small pieces of cheese or hot dog to mark your trail. Make sure pieces of any food are very small, to keep Fido from feeling full or getting too many calories. (Make sure that when you add treats to a dog's daily diet, you reduce the quantity of regular food he receives by a proportionate amount.) As you walk, toss the treats ahead, on the ground in front of the dog (we know someone who shoots them way ahead with a slingshot). Treat walks are a joyful adventure for any dog from time to time (how about one on your pooch's birthday or during National Pet Week the first week in May?), and they're an effective way to motivate dogs who aren't inclined to keep up.

2. The Doggie-Gamble Game

SLOT machines don't pay off every time they're played, and neither should you. Just as a $5 jackpot will quicken the pulse of some winners while others need a $1,000 payout to start dancing, so, too, do dogs vary in what it takes to get them to play the walking game. Treat your dog to the anticipation that you might pull a delectable morsel out at any time. Then, at irregular intervals, actually give him the thrill of victory by opening your hand to provide a piece of some-

HANSEL AND GRETEL FOR THE POKEY POOCH . . .

For a dog who lags behind, praise any forward movement as your dog goes after the treats on the trail, and don't pull on the leash. Gradually increase the distance from treat to treat, then begin giving treats from your hand as you walk backward. No pulling! Praise loose-lead walking and soon your dog will be following along behind you with the hopeful, joyful attitude you can't help but love. Once you've got your dog's interest, incorporate the Doggie-Gamble Game to keep him interested and cooperative—but not overstuffed!

thing your pet considers a jackpot. Some pets, like Dr. Becker's golden retriever, Shakira, would get excited about eating a piece of cardboard as long as their owner was excited about giving it to them. For Shakira, a baby carrot or a nugget of regular dog food is enough. Other dogs have more discriminating tastes: the Becker family's papillon/poodle/Yorkie cross, Quixote, needs a piece of hot dog, liverwurst, or freeze-dried meat to make his eyes light up. Regardless of your dog's attitude toward what you're offering, act happy and excited as you give any treat.

3. Speak Your Dog's Language

EVEN with a food bribe, not every dog is easily motivated to come to you when you're standing and holding the other end of the leash. In that case, try this: get down on your knees, then slap your thighs and speak in a high-pitched baby-talk voice to your dog (and hope

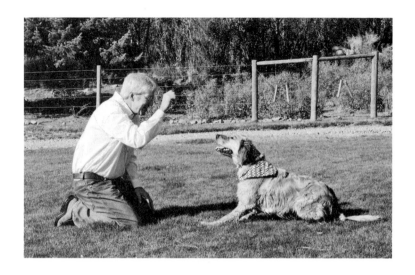

no one is watching). Getting down low makes you more attractive, and slapping at your legs mimics what behaviorists call the Play Bow that dogs do as a come-on to potential playmates. Dogs, with their rears in the air, paw the ground with their front feet, which means, "I want to be your friend—come play with me!" For most dogs, this maneuver has an almost magnetic pull that will bring them toward you for praise and petting. Once you get that go-ahead, move back to the end of the leash again, and repeat. Once your dog gets the idea, you can just lean down, and he'll follow. Dogs are natural Zen Buddhists in that they live in the moment, so it's important to reward the behavior you want as it happens. Be sure you accompany this exercise with lots of enthusiasm and encouragement.

4. Heap Praise

WOULD your pet rather perform on his own *American Idol* for Simon Scowl or Paula Abdrool? There's no contest. As far as dogs are concerned, most people are too stingy with encouragement. Let your cup runneth over with praise. Your pet will respond best if you are happy and effusive. Make your dog's first baby steps on the leash and his tail-dragging last lap around the block extra-special by heaping on a load of "good girl's" and "atta-boy's." If you consistently dole out the sweet talk and cheering on during walk times, your dog will quickly learn to respond and look forward to the pleasant "conversation" of your excursions together, too.

5. Dogs Just Want to Have Fun

WHAT do they use to train bomb- or drug-sniffing police and military dogs? A treat? Baby talk? No, they use the promise of play, often in the form of a tennis ball or a Kong toy. And that promise works equally well regardless of breed, from the smart and serious to the flaky and fun. The sight of a tennis ball gets Shakira so excited she's like a furry teapot that's building up steam and ready to blow. When you're walking, try keeping a favorite toy in your pocket or pack. At random (both time and place) pull it out and be a pet playmate. The possibility of an impromptu session of his favorite game will make him all the more enthusiastic and cooperative on the walk.

6. Let Your Dog Lead

TO bond strongly with your dog, take one walk a week in which you let him lead while you follow behind. You'll discover how your dog thinks, what interests him, and how the amazing canine senses work by observing what catches his eyes, ears, and nose in nature and in the neighborhood. For some dogs it may be a particular squirrel by a particular tree that flips their "on" switch; others may love to take their time and luxuriate in the smells that permeate a particular path; still others may love walks near the woods, where creatures communicate in ways that are as riveting to them as *Desperate Housewives* or the Super Bowl is to us.

7. Rechargeable Batteries Included!

FACE IT, our pets are pleasure beggars. They root at our hands as we sit, scratch our faces in bed, and rub up against us at every opportunity in an effort to get us to pet, scratch, rub, and massage their backs, bellies, and ears. While you're walking, pat your dog on the head or reach down and stroke his back, and he'll likely quicken the pace like an Iditarod dog on the outskirts of Nome. If your dog seems to be running out of steam, stop, take a break, and reward him with a quick massage. For many dogs, it'll seem like you just put new batteries in as they light up and get ready to take off again.

8. Alter Your Pace

ARDEN MOORE, author of more than a dozen books on dogs, including *Tricks & Games* and *Healthy Dog: The Ultimate Fitness Guide for You and Your Dog*, recommends varying your pace from slow to fast and back again to keep your dog's attention and interest on a walk. If you're still working on basic leash manners with your dog, try using a switchback route (rather than one that just goes straight forward). Altering your direction periodically helps focus your dog's attention on keeping pace with you and letting you lead the way.

9. The More the Merrier

DOGS aren't loners, they're pack animals. And while you are certainly a member of your dog's pack, you're not capable of sniffing the sidewalk and smelling the bird that walked across it five minutes ago or answering the baying dog that's calling out to Rover from a distant household. If your dog enjoys the company of other dogs, invite someone to bring another dog and walk with you. Make sure the dogs meet on neutral territory. Let your dog see you greet the other dog. Keep the leashes loose, and act happy and jolly when they first meet. Not only will dogs share their outdoor experiences and sensory world with a bosom buddy, they'll be eager to repeat the rendezvous.

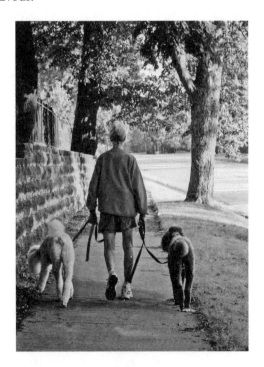

10. Road Trip

WHEN you want to drive from Point A to Point B fast, you take a direct route. When you want to relax or feel adventuresome, you take a new route or the long way. It's the same for a walk with your dog. Mix it up! Change your routes. Visit new neighborhoods and parks. Rather than walking linearly, think about meandering and exposing your dog (and yourself) to new sights and scents. Your pet needs intellectual stimulation almost as much as basic exercise, and there are few better ways to provide it than by giving him a whole new environment to think about.

You'll be repaid for every extra bit of energy you expend to engage your dog on your walks together—both in his enthusiasm to walk with you and in the benefits you'll both reap as you lose weight and gain health.

CHAPTER 8

Roadblocks and Setbacks

If losing weight were easy, there wouldn't be so many methods and programs and plans designed to help people do it successfully. With all the catchy books, high-energy DVDs, hypnotic CDs, exotic supplements, and unusual contraptions available, you'd think you'd have all the tools you need to rebuild a better body. While we believe that Fitness Unleashed offers a better chance of success than almost any other program or product out there (and certainly has unique rewards in keeping both pets and people physically fit and emotionally healthy), it's important to accept that obstacles and setbacks are inevitable as you begin. Instead of viewing them as interruptions in the program, consider them a part of it—new challenges that push you to persevere and succeed.

Ever see a dog drop out of an important chase (another dog, a squirrel, a treat) at the first obstacle? No, and neither should you. You need to go into this program with the mind-set of someone who will fly over speed bumps, blast through roadblocks, avoid trapdoors, and seek out blazed trails but not get put off by the occasional detour. In this chapter, you'll find a number of problems our patients and clients have often encountered in the past, along with the advice we've given to help them work through those issues and keep progressing.

Fear of Failure

OVER the years we've met many, many people who've had bad experiences with weight-loss programs. They've made radical diet changes or worked themselves to the bone at the gym, only to discover that what they accomplished wasn't sustainable in the long run. The reason, of course, is that it's incredibly difficult to completely change your lifestyle all at once and stick with those changes forever. A lifetime of habits—good and bad, healthy and not so healthy—doesn't fall to the wayside because you lose 10 pounds on a fad diet or in any other temporary situation any more than when you lose 10 pounds because you've had the flu. Eventually you feel "normal" again and your lifestyle comes full circle.

Many of the folks we know who have experienced this kind of disappointment come away with a "Why bother?" attitude or with the feeling that they are doomed to failure at the outset of any weight-loss or fitness program.

With Fitness Unleashed, we encourage small, sustainable changes to your lifestyle—never a full, sweeping, extreme makeover. The biggest of these is simply making the commitment to spend quality time with your dog by walking together a few times a week, increasing the duration and intensity of those walks over time. There's a good chance you'll be able to see, hear, and feel how much this benefits your dog even before you can feel the benefits yourself—a great motivator for any dog owner to stick with the program.

The second component to Fitness Unleashed is the nutritional changes we recommend. These are small changes that you choose to commit to one week at a time. There's never a moment when you must vow to give up sugar, or snacks, or butter, or bread, or hamburgers forever. Instead, if you consider the recommendations for your eating pattern in Chapter 3 and choose your mini-goals each week from Chapter 6 (page 156), you'll find that these small changes work with, not against, your lifestyle.

Nothing's Happening!

IT'S frustrating to make changes (even small ones) in your routine and then find they don't produce the desired results. Unfortunately, it's all too common to take on a program, give it two weeks, then give up. Please don't! Everyone's body loses weight in its own way. We can't tell you how many times we've worked with clients who stick with a program for ten days, think they've gotten nowhere, then "suddenly" find they've lost 5 pounds. Instead of placing too much "weight" on the scale reading, try to judge by the way you feel, by how your clothes fit, and by whether you've been faithfully increas-

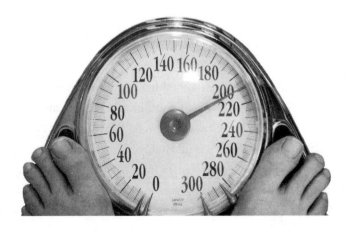

DOG TIME

A setback in your own routine is bad enough, but when it means your dog is going to lose out on his workout, too, well, that's an even bigger bummer. Dogs are remarkably loving and forgiving, so if you've got to forego a walk—or a series of walks—for any reason, be sure to give your dog some extra time and affection (*not* extra treats) at your regular workout time to make up for it. Alternatively, get a family member or friend to walk the dog for you, or substitute an exercise for your dog such as chasing a tennis ball or swimming at a local pond until you feel like being towed around the neighborhood again.

ing your time and steps walked each week. We strongly recommend you stick to the program for a full six weeks before passing judgment on it. By then you'll be able to see results for both you and your dog.

Dealing with Sickness and Injury

THE good news is that walking is safe and poses a minimal risk of injury.

The bad news is that even something as simple and unforeseeable as a twisted ankle, a flare-up of gout, or a bad cold can leave you wanting nothing to do with a long walk. When sickness or injury happens in your life, which it inevitably will at some point, remind yourself that everyone gets sidelined from time to time, and the critical issue is about whether you'll stay in control of your lifestyle.

When you're sick or injured, broaden your focus from thinking about weight to thinking about your health in general. Give your body a chance to heal and rest, and know that by doing so you are still in control of your eating and activity level: you're wisely choosing rest over exercise so you can look forward to getting back on track when you're well again. Speaking of "on track," racing greyhounds that are injured stay "off the track" until they're healed. Never try to force a sick or injured dog to walk before he's cleared by the veterinarian.

As you do feel better and healthier, ease back to your previous level (one week earlier than where you left off) in the Fitness Unleashed program, rather than jumping right back in where you were beforehand. If you need to go back to the beginning, that's fine. If you've been very ill or badly hurt, you'll benefit from the fresh air and the time spent exercising with your dog. A little walk will help inspire you to take a longer one when you're ready.

Too Busy, Too Tired, or Too Depressed

WE accept, and you should, too, that there are times in your life when you can't keep up with your exercise routine, or when your eating habits get away from you and you feel like you may never get back your control. When this happens to you, make a decision to carry on some part of the program (even if it's just the mini-goals for a few days) or to do a specific portion of your walking routine (for example, commit to doing half this week and going back to "full-time" in the next; or keep wearing your pedometer, because it may inspire you to add steps in other areas to help compensate for lost walks). We want you to feel consistently that your eating choices and exercise efforts are matters of your choice—that you are in control of your lifestyle and schedule. There's nothing at all wrong with giving yourself a break from time to time.

Gaining Back Weight

FIRST and foremost, don't panic. Weight plateaus and gaining back weight are almost always as much a part of the process of losing it as taking the pounds off for good. We'd like you to think of Fitness Unleashed (or any weight-loss program, for that matter) not as a long walk down a straight road toward your goal, but rather as a dance step that moves a few steps forward, and then a couple steps back. This is the reality of any long-term success, and you'll benefit a great deal from looking at any pound that creeps back on—or any weight-loss plateaus—as an integral part of the process and not a sign that you've done something wrong.

Stick to the program. Add a few minutes to each of your walks. You'll be back on track before you know it.

Holidays, Vacations, and Other Sitting-Around-and-Eating Occasions

THE last thing we want you to do on Fitness Unleashed is suffer through a holiday, a vacation, or a party feeling deprived. This program is about feeling great and about helping your dog to feel great, too. Give yourself permission to enjoy the foods and occasions you love, and simply practice moderation. If at all possible, continue to take your walks, continue to wear your pedometer, and choose two simple mini-goals to keep in mind during these times.

At the Wellness Institute, Dr. Kushner encourages his patients to make weight maintenance—not necessarily loss—their goal over the holidays. This is a smart, realistic approach for any special occasion for you, too.

My Dog Doesn't Want to Walk!

YES, this happens, though not very often. If your dog doesn't want to walk, there are a few possible reasons. Never fear, each can be overcome with a little patience and practice.

- A health problem. Occasionally, an issue like arthritis, an infection, sore foot pads, or a metabolic problem such as low thyroid can contribute to a dog not wanting to walk. Please make an appointment with your dog's veterinarian to make sure any of these issues is diagnosed and treated.
- Fear. A fearful dog may give you subtle (or not so subtle) signs that he's not comfortable getting outside and exploring. Behaviors range from a dog licking its lips, yawning, scratching, or avoiding eye contact with you to shrinking away or hiding. Fear may show in ambivalent behavior, such as when the dog seems to want to go outside with you but also acts

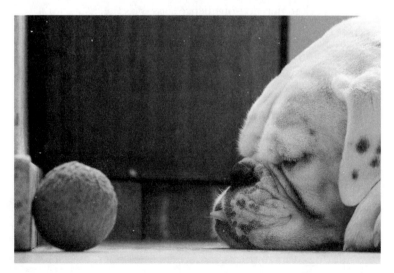

anxious. In more severe cases, your dog may tremble, cower, tuck his tail between his legs, or run away when you get ready to take him for a walk.

If this sounds like your dog, don't force him to suddenly face his fears—odds are that tactic will only make them worse. Comforting your dog—even though it comes naturally to you—is also a common mistake, as it unintentionally reinforces and may increase the fear. Instead, help your dog overcome his fears by building his confidence in gentle progressive steps—small, indirect exposures to the things that scare him. If you need help, a qualified animal behaviorist can guide you through this desensitization process. You can also find professional help at www.animalbehavior.net.

The three most common fears related to leash walking are fear of the leash itself, noise phobias, and a condition behaviorists call neophobia, or fear of things that are new.

Leash fear and avoidance may be the easiest to explain. Think back to that dog-obedience class. Was the instructor a cross between a drill sergeant and a hangman? Did you or someone else attempt to leash-train your dog less than gently when he was a puppy? If so, your dog may associate the leash with being jerked around by the neck. He may believe that now, every time the leash is snapped on, he's heading back to boot camp. Alternatively, it may be that your dog just never got used to the leash in the first place. If either of these is the case, purchase a new leash, and begin the leash-training program described in Chapter 5 to help your dog get past his fear and start walking happily beside you.

A phobia is an excessive and unnecessary fear reaction. Some dogs react to trucks, motorcycles, and hot rods as if they were fire-breathing dragons. If your dog suffers from one of these common fears, try taking him to a very quiet place for peaceful walks. (If you live in the city, you might have to take a few car trips to the country, for example.) If your dog's phobia is other dogs or bicycles or strange men—anything he commonly encounters on your outings—try a similar approach. Find a place where your dog can have a pleasant walk—without facing his fear—and then work your way back to your normal walk once he's become confident in the sheltered environment.

Neophobia means "fear of the unknown." This might include fear of the leash itself as well as everything outside. To prevent neophobia, most veterinarians now recommend puppy-socialization classes for puppies two to four months old. If you have an adult dog who suffers from this problem, you're going to have to be patient and help your dog adjust to the outside world one small step at a time. For this dog, choose the quietest, least congested route you can find, and stick with the same place, gradually increasing your walk time, while your dog becomes confident with the venue.

The "nosy" dog. If your dog is too busy sniffing every corner, you can't get the exercise you both need. This is especially common in male dogs who are not neutered as well as in certain hunting breeds such as beagles. Once they get used to the leash, many dogs want nothing more than to sniff and pee, sniff and pee—not exactly the pace you're hoping to establish to raise your heart rate and burn calories.

The key to keeping your dog on the move is to decide how many stops you're willing to allow and when. If your dog needs to relieve himself, that should be a guaranteed stop. If he's decided to "water" every tree or mailbox, well, that's just not the same. Establish a signal from the very beginning of your walking program that means "We're not stopping here" and stick with it. A phrase like "Leave it" or "Let's go" will fill the bill. Use an extendable leash, which allows Fido to run ahead or lag behind and have a sniffing moment without holding you up. As you reach the end of the leash in either case, though, clearly speak your "Let's go" phrase and keep walking. At first, this may result in some neck pulling (though not neck jerking) with the leash. If you're consistent with the timing of the command and the moment of moving forward at the end of the leash, though, your dog will quickly figure out that you mean what you say.

Walking without sniffing isn't nearly as much fun for your dog as walking with it. Once he understands "Let's go" or the other phrase you've chosen to convey that it's time to move forward, you can add another phrase to your conversations—one that allows your dog to take an extra minute to smell something that fascinates him. Choose a phrase like "Take a sniff," or "I'll wait" (something that does not sound like your "Let's go" phrase). When your dog is really fascinated with a smell, give him the okay with the "Take a sniff" phrase, wait for a minute or two, then use your "Let's go" and be on your way. Your dog will appreciate the chance to stop and have extra smelling time now and then, and you'll still be in control of when and how often he makes his sniffing stops.

● Wandering. If your dog just doesn't seem inclined to keep moving, and if he doesn't show any signs of being tired or distressed, it's time to introduce the one gadget more savvy dog walkers, animal behaviorists, and pet trainers swear by than any other we know. The product known as a Gentle Leader Headcollar can help resolve almost any walking-related problem with a dog. The head collar will not hurt your dog, but it will compel him to let you be the "driver" on your walks because it corrects him in the same way (with pressure at the top of his nose) that a mother dog would. Once you help your dog overcome the behavior that's been disrupting your walks, the head collar converts to a regular collar. (More information about the harness and how it works appears in Chapter 5.)

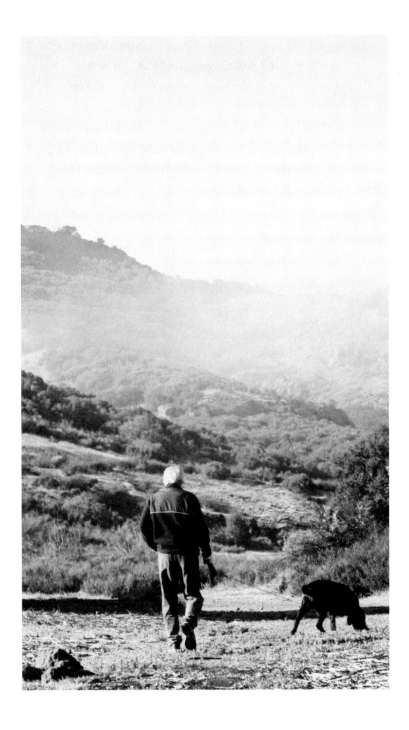

CHAPTER 9

Success!

Success in unleashing fitness comes in many different forms: pounds lost, strength gained, an elated walker, relationships with neighbors you'd previously shared a street with but never a conversation, a happy pet, an enriched bond between you and your dog—sometimes even a piece of furniture that gets a reprieve from the chewing of a previously pent-up pooch. We'd like to share the stories of a few of the many wonderful people we've met and interviewed who have taken the simple idea of walking the dog and made big changes in their weight, their health, and their level of enjoyment of everyday life. They've been an inspiration to us as we write about the wealth of benefits of Fitness Unleashed.

Scaling Down

MAGGIE MORGAN, of West Michigan, is a wife, a mom, a teacher, and a dog owner. For most of her adult life, she's made fitness a priority by eating healthy foods, playing tennis, and even teaching aerobics. But a few years ago, she found her routine slipping and 30 unwanted pounds gradually crept onto her frame.

Getting active again was a priority, but it wasn't easy for Maggie, who describes herself as phobic about exercising in public. She started her weight-loss program in the dead of winter, pounding away at home on a treadmill in her basement, not losing any weight, but not gaining any either. She joined Dr. Kushner's online weight-loss community at diet.com and found reassurance and inspiration in setting mini-goals and being reminded that successfully dropping pounds requires lifestyle changes you abide by for the long term—not just a couple weeks. When spring rolled around, Maggie wanted to be able to stretch her legs, enjoy some sun, and even run, and she looked to her dogs, a golden retriever named Holly and a beagle called Snoopy, to help her make the adjustment from exercising in the privacy of her own home to getting outdoors and facing the world. "When I walk past someone with one of my dogs, they detract all the attention from me, because they're so darned cute," she explains. "They're like a canine shield."

They're also an inspiration to start walking and keep walking. "I would much rather walk with a dog than alone," Maggie explains, "They love the fresh air, the neighbors, and the wildlife, and they adapt to any pace I set."

Maggie's pace has picked up substantially since she started walking. Both she and the dogs needed to take some time to build up their endurance, but these days they intersperse segments of jogging with their walks. Maggie has lost 19 pounds in her quest to regain fitness, striving to exercise for 45 minutes on most days. Snoopy has lost 3 pounds and his veterinarian declared him the first beagle he's seen in a long time who's not overweight. Holly, the golden retriever, continues to maintain her weight, but she's become more energetic, less easily winded, and able to walk longer distances.

ITALIAN DOGS DON'T GET FAT

At least not those in Rome, thanks to a piece of legislation passed in early 2005. According to the law, pet owners are required to walk their dogs at least three times a day. Not doing so can result in a fine of up to five hundred euros (about six hundred dollars). Due to the threat of the steep fines looming, we like to think of this particular "program," which is bound to influence human fitness along with that of dogs', as Fitness Unleashed—Or Else.

A Little Canine Inspiration

FOR most women, coming home with a new baby means beginning a period of rest, recovery, and figuring out how best to love and care for an infant. For Teri Sue Wright, a veterinarian in Eugene, Oregon, and a new mother with just about forty-eight hours of parenting experience under her belt, it meant returning home to find two stir-crazy dogs who desperately wanted a walk.

She might have been inclined to pass the dogs by on the way to the couch, but Dr. Wright couldn't ignore the excitement of her Labrador retriever, Pilot, and her Chesapeake Bay retriever, Taz, for a number of good reasons. First, she was already looking forward to picking up her exercise routine and losing the weight she'd gained during the pregnancy. Second, it was a pretty day in the Pacific Northwest, and the dogs did seem to have a point about the wisdom of getting outside. And most of all, there was Taz's sheer will to go. Months before, Dr. Wright had brought Taz home from her veterinary practice for rehabilitation after the dog had had one paw amputated. Taz had been a guard dog, and when she was no longer able to work, her owner didn't want her anymore. Despite the pain and

MAN'S BEST (BATTERY-OPERATED) FRIEND?

If a group of researchers at the Massachusetts Institute of Technology has their way, many people who can't have or don't want dogs will soon be able to share in one of the health benefits that comes with canine companionship. The scientists are working on a robotic dog that will remind its owner when it's time for scheduled exercise. In addition, the virtual pet will use a radio link to the owner's pedometer, bathroom scale, and personal organizer (which would ideally contain a food diary) to help keep tabs on calories consumed, steps walked, and weight. When asked a weight loss–related question like "How am I doing?" by the owner, the robot will deliver a response based on that data: a funny dance and bright lights for the owner who has stuck to the plan or lost weight, or lying down and looking miserable for the one who has gained or fallen off the wagon.

discomfort of her injury, Taz seemed to relish the opportunity to just be a silly around-the-house dog for a change. And even though her foot had to be bandaged and covered with a plastic bag for each walk, she was eager to go at every opportunity.

"The day I came home with the baby, it probably took me ten minutes to get Taz ready to go, and another ten to get the baby wrapped up and tucked into the sling, but it felt great to be outside and walking again after being in the hospital," Dr. Wright remembers. Within a couple of weeks, she had resumed her forty-five-minutes-a-day, five days-a-week walking routine, and by the time she was eight weeks postpartum, the walks had gently and steadily helped her lose all the baby weight.

"I'm actually thinner now than I was when I got pregnant," Dr. Wright says. "I've got to give a lot of the credit to the dogs. Day after day, they just make me feel like I have to go. I hate to let them down."

Rediscovering the Great Outdoors

LIZ Luisi grew up as an outdoorsy girl, spending her summer days on the shores of Cape Cod. As an adult, Liz shared her love of nature and fresh air with her family, frequently taking long walks, having picnics, and planning hiking outings. Then two years ago, Liz got sick and didn't seem to be able to get better. After months of feeling exhausted and coping with joint pain and frequent bladder infections, she was diagnosed with Lyme disease—an estimated eight months after she first got it. She began a long treatment with antibiotics that made her feel even more weak and tired.

"I never even knew there was a tick," Liz says. "After I was diagnosed, and for months while I was taking the antibiotics, I really felt afraid to do anything outdoors." Not only did Liz not want to spend time outside herself, but she also didn't want her kids to be out any more than necessary. She felt as though everyone she loved was in danger of getting sick, too.

The strain of her sickness and anxiety started to turn around when Liz's stepson, Andrew, finally convinced the family that it was time to get a dog. After Andrew promised to train the dog himself, and after several family debates about what breed would be suitable, the Luisis welcomed a black Labrador retriever puppy named Bella.

Getting the dog, Liz explains, became a turning point in her treatment. "I was really sick and weak and stuck inside, and along comes this puppy who needs to get out and who takes so much joy in experiencing the world. It forced me to get outside, and I kind of had the opportunity to start fresh with her."

Starting fresh has included ventures ranging from trips around the block on the sidewalk to Liz's first trip since her diagnosis back to Cape Cod to visit her family. "I would have been really afraid to be out on the beach, but Bella was running out to the water and chasing it and having such a blast, I was able to enjoy it. Having her in our lives hasn't eliminated my fear that someone in my family could get a tick and get sick, but it has helped me put that fear in perspective."

The Luisi family's timely acquisition of a dog is also helping Liz to build up her strength after more than a year of sickness. She and Bella are just beginning to start a walking program together, and Liz is looking forward to it for both of them. "We're both going to bene-fit from the exercise," she says. "I'm walking for the first time in a long time, and it's been really good to feel a little stronger again. I've been able to do it because Bella needs it and she's with me. I'm really grateful to be able to be even thinking about fitness again, and this dog has made a huge contribution to that."

Behavior Management with a Side of Fitness

AT least twice a week, it's bring-your-dog-to-work day at the offices of Greeley and Associates in Spokane, Washington. Those are the days when David Greeley, M.D., a neurologist with a busy practice, brings his two-year-old Irish terrier, Finnegan, to the office. Dr. Greeley started bringing Finnegan because the dog needed an outlet for more of his energy. "My wife and I have three girls, and we're both busy, and there were days when the dog was at home and just acting like a crazy kid wanting to know what he could possibly get into next."

Of course, a dog with boundless energy doesn't mix well in an of-fice environment, either. To get Finnegan ready for his days at the of-fice, Dr. Greeley started taking him for a run. "I probably ran five times a year before we had a dog," he laughs, "but now I run twice a week, on the days I bring Finn to the office. The dog loves it so much

I can't help but go. I often start to think that I don't really enjoy running—until I'm out there, and then I realize it's much more enjoyable and rewarding than sitting around reading the newspaper, after all."

Dr. Greeley modestly describes himself as having been "one of those guys who's five foot ten and weighs 150 pounds wet" when he started running regularly with Finnegan. He has been surprised and pleased to find that the new routine has improved his muscle tone, his ability to sleep well at night, and his energy level. Since he was very thin to begin with, he's actually been able to add about 5 pounds of muscle since running, a welcome addition to his lean frame.

"It's kind of odd, because as a doctor I always tell my patients that getting regular exercise is one of the very best things they can do for their own health," he muses, "but as a busy professional, it was very hard for me to put that into practice myself. Now, Finnegan just makes me go, and we're both happier and healthier for it."

For the Love of a Dog

FOR some dogs, a 40-minute-walk is nothing but a warmup—and almost any one-year-old Labrador retriever you can find fits into that category. It is certainly true of Winston, the fourteen-month-old Lab who belongs to Jack and Sandra McBride of Colfax, Washington. What sets the McBrides apart from many people who own big, energetic, adolescent dogs is that Jack and Sandy are not just waiting out this phase of dog developement. They didn't choose this puppy because they wanted a mellow, hearth rug–loving dog . They chose him because they knew he'd contribute to their healthy lifestyles by giving them even more incentive to exercise.

Jack consistently strives to maintain a rigorous exercise program. He's always been athletic, even running three marathons in years past, but he had concerns that he might not be as active in his retirement. With the addition of Winston to the household, that very quickly became a nonissue. Jack and Winston walk forty-five minutes to an hour every day—about four miles total. After Sandy, who's a nurse, comes home from work, they sometimes walk again. On Sandy's days off, the couple often bikes several miles along a rural road to a stream, with Winston gleefully running alongside them until his favorite moment—the one when he dives into the water to cool off and splash around.

"I definitely believe that Winston has been a godsend to Sandy and me," Jack says. "We're both concerned about our health, and we both benefit from the extra motivation Winston brings. If he was not here, I know I wouldn't be going so consistently. But I have a dog who appreciates and needs the exercise, and that's plenty of motivation to keep me going day after day."

A PPET Success

WHEN Kathleen O'Dekirk first met Dr. Kushner in 2002, she had two very compelling reasons to give a new approach to weight loss a try: First, the five-foot-three-inch, forty-nine-year-old attorney had just bought her first pair of size 14 pants and was none too happy about it. Second, Kathleen's dog, Winston (no relation to the Winston above!), had gone from solid to chubby to dangerously tubby and both Kathleen and her dog's veterinarian were worried about his health. Winston, a Cavalier King Charles spaniel, should have weighed in near the breed standard of 18 pounds—maybe a little heavier, because he's tall for the breed. Instead, Winston was waddling around at 31 pounds—and no amount of height or big bones could account for that much excess baggage.

Like so many of us who've broken down and given in to buying bigger pants, Kathleen wasn't sure how she'd gone from rail thin in her twenties to panicking about having to jump up yet another size as she contemplated her fiftieth birthday. "When I reached thirty, I put on a little weight," she says. "At thirty-five, I put on a little more. By the time I was in my mid-forties, all the little gains had become a big problem. I didn't really feel like I was eating too much, but I'd reached the point where my legs and my back hurt when Winston and I walked to the coffee shop five blocks away. I was uncomfortable, and I was coming up on that milestone birthday, and ready to do something different."

Kathleen couldn't pinpoint Winston's weight-gain problem either. She'd cut back on his snacks and changed his food, but he continued to put on pounds.

When Kathleen saw a blurb in the *Chicago Tribune* about a research study seeking overweight people with overweight dogs, she called and signed up to participate in People and Pets Exercising Together. She'll be the first to tell you that dropping 14 pounds and two sizes during the study, which she did, was hard work, and also that incorporating the walking recommendations of the study was the first step on her road to fitness. "I thought Winston and I were already walkers," Kathleen claims. "When I started steadily increasing our steps and monitoring them with the pedometer, I realized we could do much more.

"At first, my eating habits didn't change at all. I was writing down everything I ate, though, so my food log would say things like, 'Fried chicken, gravy, and corn bread.' The more and longer Winston and I walked, though, the better I felt, and the more I was open to looking at my food choices, too."

As for Winston, with the help of a prescription diet food from Hill's Pet Nutrition and frequent long walks, he whittled away 7 pounds and today acts like he's aged backward from the heavy (and heavy-breathing) dog he was just three years ago.

Today, Kathleen and Winston walk an hour or more a day, and Winston would prefer to go even farther if Kathleen would let him. They are both fit and trim and healthy. "The study helped show me what I had to do to take control of my body and my health," she says. "It was a great step for me and a wonderful turning point for Winston."

We hope you'll come away from *Fitness Unleashed* with a new appreciation of the health benefits you and your dog can achieve together. Your dog does need you to help him achieve and maintain good health, but in return for doing so, he can take on the role of motivator, exercise partner, and all-around cheering section in your commitment to exercise. The benefits of getting up and out and sticking to a regular, challenging walking routine do include weight loss, but they also go well beyond it—to everything from decreased risk of cancer, heart disease, and Alzheimer's to strengthened and toned muscles and an appreciation of a new neighbor or the beauty of the great outdoors.

We wish you good health, a strengthened bond with your dog, a joyful experience in exercise, and much success as you and your dog set out to lose weight, gain health, and unleash fitness together.

appendix

Additional Recommended Resources

BOOKS:

Dr. Kushner's Personality Type Diet by Robert Kushner, M.D., and
   Nancy Kushner, M.S.N., R.N.
The Healing Power of Pets by Dr. Marty Becker with Danelle Morton

WEBSITES:

www.diet.com: Dr. Kushner's personalized online weight-loss program using a
   validated personality test, customized weight-loss strategies, meal plans, and
   social support.
www.doctorkushner.com: Dr. Kushner's website.
www.drmartybecker.com: Dr. Becker's website.
www.hikewithyourdog.com: A great site with info and links for more than 2,000
   dog-friendly places to hike and walk.
www.dog-play.com: All kinds of activities you can do with your dog, including
   specific locations across the United States.
www.animalplanet.com: If you click on the section called "Pet Guides & Tools,"
   you'll find, among other resources, the "Dog Parks USA" link. It features an
   interactive map of dog parks.

HEALTH AND FITNESS ORGANIZATIONS:

American Animal Hospital
Association
www.healthypet.com
1-800-883-6301

Arthritis Foundation
www.arthritis.org
1-800-568-4045

American Cancer Society
www.cancer.org

American College of Sports
Medicine
www.acsm.org

American Council on Exercise
www.acefitness.org
1-800-825-3636

American Heart Association
www.americanheart.org
1-800-AHA-USA-1

American Veterinary Medical
Association
www.avma.org

The Cooper Institute
www.cooperinst.org

Weight Watchers International
www.weightwatchers.com

Fitness Unleashed Progress Log

MY STARTING WEIGHT _____

STARTING WEIGHT THIS WEEK _____

DOG STARTING WEIGHT _____

Diet Mini-Goals: This week I will:

1 _____

2 _____

3 (optional) _____

Progress Log forms can be downloaded and printed from
www.diet.com/fitnessunleashed.

	STEPS TAKEN	WALKING TIME	PERSONAL & PET NOTES
MONDAY			
TUESDAY			
WEDNESDAY			
THURSDAY			
FRIDAY			
SATURDAY			
SUNDAY			

Last Week's Average Daily Steps _____

This Week's Average Daily Steps _____

BMI Table

BMI	19	20	21	22	23	24	25	26	27	28	29	30	31	32	33	34	35
Height (inches)	Body Weight (pounds)																
58	91	96	100	105	110	115	119	124	129	134	138	143	148	153	158	162	167
59	94	99	104	109	114	119	124	128	133	138	143	148	153	158	163	168	173
60	97	102	107	112	118	123	128	133	138	143	148	153	158	163	168	174	179
61	100	106	111	116	122	127	132	137	143	148	153	158	164	169	174	180	185
62	104	109	115	120	126	131	136	142	147	153	158	164	169	175	180	186	191
63	107	113	118	124	130	135	141	146	152	158	163	169	175	180	186	191	197
64	110	116	122	128	134	140	145	151	157	163	169	174	180	186	192	197	204
65	114	120	126	132	138	144	150	156	162	168	174	180	186	192	198	204	210
66	118	124	130	136	142	148	155	161	167	173	179	186	192	198	204	210	216
67	121	127	134	140	146	153	159	166	172	178	185	191	198	204	211	217	223
68	125	131	138	144	151	158	164	171	177	184	190	197	203	210	216	223	230
69	128	135	142	149	155	162	169	176	182	189	196	203	209	216	223	230	236
70	132	139	146	153	160	167	174	181	188	195	202	209	216	222	229	236	243
71	136	143	150	157	165	172	179	186	193	200	208	215	222	229	236	243	250
72	140	147	154	162	169	177	184	191	199	206	213	221	228	235	242	250	258
73	144	151	159	166	174	182	189	197	204	212	219	227	235	242	250	257	265
74	148	155	163	171	179	186	194	202	210	218	225	233	241	249	256	264	272
75	152	160	168	176	184	192	200	208	216	224	232	240	248	256	264	272	279
76	156	164	172	180	189	197	205	213	221	230	238	246	254	263	271	279	287

BMI	36	37	38	39	40	41	42	43	44	45	46	47	48	49	50	51	52	53	54
58	172	177	181	186	191	196	201	205	210	215	220	224	229	234	239	244	248	253	258
59	178	183	188	193	198	203	208	212	217	222	227	232	237	242	247	252	257	262	267
60	184	189	194	199	204	209	215	220	225	230	235	240	245	250	255	261	266	271	276
61	190	195	201	206	211	217	222	227	232	238	243	248	254	259	264	269	275	280	285
62	196	202	207	213	218	224	229	235	240	246	251	256	262	267	273	278	284	289	295
63	203	208	214	220	225	231	237	242	248	254	259	265	270	278	282	287	293	299	304
64	209	215	221	227	232	238	244	250	256	262	267	273	279	285	291	296	302	308	314
65	216	222	228	234	240	246	252	258	264	270	276	282	288	294	300	306	312	318	324
66	223	229	235	241	247	253	260	266	272	278	284	291	297	303	309	315	322	328	334
67	230	236	242	249	255	261	268	274	280	287	293	299	306	312	319	325	331	338	344
68	236	243	249	256	262	269	276	282	289	295	302	308	315	322	328	335	341	348	354
69	243	250	257	263	270	277	284	291	297	304	311	318	324	331	338	345	351	358	365
70	250	257	264	271	278	285	292	299	306	313	320	327	334	341	348	355	362	369	376
71	257	265	272	279	286	293	301	308	315	322	329	338	343	351	358	365	372	379	386
72	265	272	279	287	294	302	309	316	324	331	338	346	353	361	368	375	383	390	397
73	272	280	288	295	302	310	318	325	333	340	348	355	363	371	378	386	393	401	408
74	280	287	295	303	311	319	326	334	342	350	358	365	373	381	389	396	404	412	420
75	287	295	303	311	319	327	335	343	351	359	367	375	383	391	399	407	415	423	431
76	295	304	312	320	328	336	344	353	361	369	377	385	394	402	410	418	426	435	443

KNOW YOUR BMI

The days of charts designed to pinpoint "ideal body weight" or "desirable body weight" are no longer used today. A more practical measurement of overweight and obesity is this chart that offers the range for your body mass index, or BMI. BMI is calculated using a mathematical formula based on a person's height and weight. The result predicts the development of health problems related to excess weight. To determine your BMI, look down the left column to find your height (in inches) and then look across that row and find the weight that's nearest your own. Now look to the top of the column to find the number that is your BMI. For example, if you are 5'4" (64" tall) and weigh 164 pounds, then your BMI would be 28.

A BMI from 18.5 through 24.9 is desirable and healthy. The goal here is to prevent any further weight gain. A BMI from 25 through 29.9 is considered overweight and carries a slightly increased risk of weight-related health problems. A BMI of 30 or more is medically designated as obesity and carries a high risk for health-related problems. Morbid or severe obesity is regarded as a BMI of 40 or greater.

The higher the BMI, the greater the risk for developing diabetes, high blood pressure, some forms of cancer, osteoarthritis, sleep disturbances, stroke, and heart disease, among others. Although BMI compares well to the percentage of body fat, it is not a direct measurement of body fat.

Please consider one important note regarding BMI: If you are highly active and muscular, your BMI risk level may appear disproportionately high for your actual body fat percentage. If you think you might fit into this category, we recommend that you have a body-fat analysis done by either skin-fold anthropometry or bioimpedence analyses at a health club or a health-care provider's office.

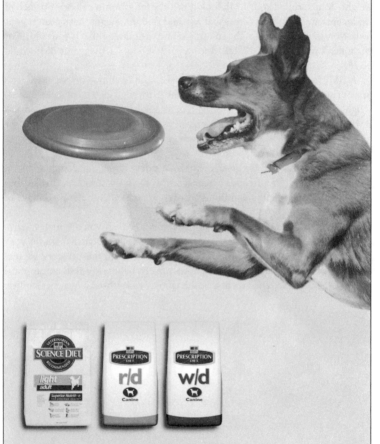

SHED UNWANTED POUNDS.
GAIN EXTRA PLAYTIME.

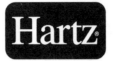
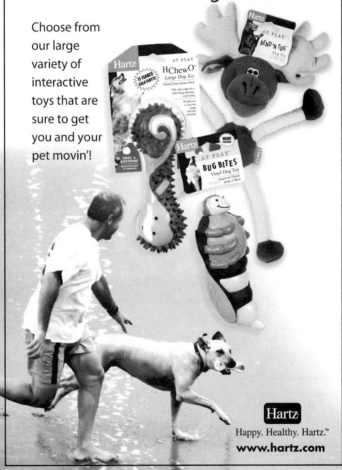

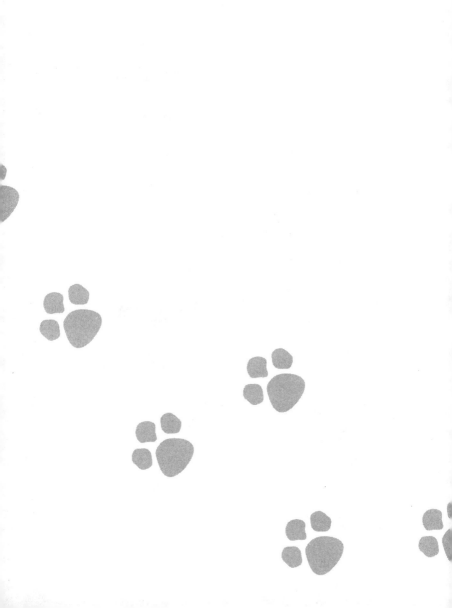